P9-DHF-328

The
Menopause
MANAGER

The
Menopause
MANAGER

A SAFE PATH
FOR A NATURAL CHANGE

Mary Ann Mayo
& Joseph L. Mayo, M.D.

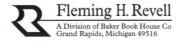

Fleming H. Revell
A Division of Baker Book House Co
Grand Rapids, Michigan 49516

© 1998 by Mary Ann Mayo and Joseph Lee Mayo

Published by Fleming H. Revell
a division of Baker Book House Company
P.O. Box 6287, Grand Rapids, MI 49516-6287

Paperback edition published 2000

Second printing, August 2000

Printed in the United States of America

All rights reserved. No part of this publication may be reproduced, stored in a retrieval system, or transmitted in any form or by any means—for example, electronic, photocopy, recording—without the prior written permission of the publisher. The only exception is brief quotations in printed reviews.

Library of Congress Cataloging-in-Publication Data

Mayo, Mary Ann.
    The menopause manager : a safe path for a natural change / Mary Ann and Joseph L. Mayo.
      p.   cm.
    Includes index.
    ISBN 0-8007-1740-6 (cloth)
    ISBN 0-8007-5733-5 (paper)
    1. Menopause—Popular works. 2. Herbs—Therapeutic use. I. Mayo, Joseph L. II. Title.
RG186.M35   1998
618.1'75—DC21   97-20700

Scripture quotations are taken from the HOLY BIBLE, NEW INTERNATIONAL VERSION®. NIV®. Copyright © 1973, 1978, 1984 by International Bible Society. Used by permission of Zondervan Publishing House. All rights reserved.

The poem in chapter 21 is used by permission of the author.

Overcaring, FREEZE FRAME, and *Cut Thru,* used in chapter 15, are registered trademarks of HeartMath.

Joseph L. Mayo, M.D., and Mary Ann Mayo, M.A., have written this book as an educational resource, not a tool to be used for diagnosis and treatment. The information presented is in no way a substitute for consultation with an individual's physician. Although the authors have carefully researched all sources to ensure the accuracy and completeness of the information, the publisher and authors shall have neither liability nor responsibility to any person or entity with respect to any loss, damage, or injury caused or alleged to be caused directly or indirectly by the information presented. Treatment of medical conditions and wellness should always be supervised by a physician or licensed health care professional.

For current information about all releases from Baker Book House, visit our web site:
http://www.bakerbooks.com

Dedicated to our mothers

Mary Jo Manahan
Frances L. Mayo

Contents

List of Figures

Foreword

Today's midlife woman may be perplexed to find herself moving through a major life passage about which she has no choice. However, once she's on her way, she is not about to leave this new and unprecedented experience to chance. After all, women of her generation did not sit quietly while their physicians medicated them into oblivion during childbirth. Nor did these women permit the fathers of their about-to-be-born babies to participate by warming a chair in front of the waiting room TV set. This woman works, reads labels, buys supplements at the health food store, takes care of her aging parents, and mothers two teenagers and a six-year-old. She is busy and she is smart. She doesn't need additional rhetoric or more philosophizing—she needs a manager: The Menopause Manager.

The information found in *The Menopause Manager* is cutting edge. It reveals endless possibilities but allows each reader to individualize her choices according to her liking and her particular requirements. Most women today are concerned about supporting their health as naturally as possible but are not ready to turn their back on the whole of conventional medicine. Yet many of the current books take an either/or approach to alternatives. *The Menopause Manager* balances medical knowledge with botanical wisdom, offering the best of both worlds.

In our experience, the women most apt to seek help with menopause are bright, active superachievers. Their chief complaint is that they aren't able to function emotionally and physically with the same focused drive that has propelled them through life thus far. Concise information, presented logically and clearly, is what they deserve and what they respond to. But they must also learn that midlife is a time when other health issues become as impor-

11

tant as menopause itself. The accurate diagnosis of everything that is going on ensures correct and effective treatment. A shift in emphasis from cure to prevention is essential, since a woman's health risk escalates at menopause.

After reading *The Menopause Manager,* a woman will understand her personal risk factors and, if necessary, the treatment options available. She will be empowered and will make medical decisions with confidence and hope. When she visits her doctor, she will expect to be taken seriously. Most important, she will see this menopause passage as a time of transition, leading to new, exciting, and healthful ways to spend the next one-third of her life.

Acknowledgments

A number of years ago just about the time I began experiencing my first signs of menopause, a publisher contacted Dr. Mayo and me to write a book about menopause. We turned them down. At the time, so little was known about women's midlife that the idea of perpetuating the guesses, assumptions, and male ivory-tower view was of no benefit to anyone—especially the women who were looking for answers. How times have changed! Knowledge has escalated scientifically, experientially, and personally. Menopause has catapulted to the forefront by numbers alone (an estimated forty million American women are now in or past menopause, another twenty million, the baby boomer generation, will reach that stage of life in the next decade—one every seven and one-half seconds for the next ten years) and by women's increasing role in medicine and in all walks of life.

When we moved from the clinic that Dr. Mayo had been associated with for almost twenty years to a solo practice specializing in midlife women, it resulted in a relocation far more profound than a mere change of address. Our new office, first in Sebastopol, California, and then down the road in Healdsburg, placed us in the heart of complementary medicine. We had access to some of the world's authorities as teachers and found ourselves challenged by patients whose experiences and knowledge pushed our learning curve to the edge. As we sifted and sorted through the amalgam of medical knowledge and botanical wisdom, a new approach to menopause evolved. A melding occurred.

There is no argument that the power to feel better and experience greater wellness, no matter in what stage of life, lies chiefly within each individual. Choices about nutrition, lifestyle, and one's spiritual outlook all impact health. Distinguishing between risk factors and symptoms provides direction. An informed decision about one's health implies commitment to make it work.

"Relocation" personally, professionally, and philosophically has been a challenge but profoundly rewarding. A Woman's Place Medical Center is not an ivory tower; it is a working clinic visited by real women, not statistics. It is from and for those women *The Menopause Manager: A Safe Path for a Natural Change* has been developed. The women's stories in the book are entirely fictional and represent composite characters only. Thanks to the real women in our lives, however, for keeping our feet on the ground and occasionally to the fire.

Thanks are due to the genuinely good people at Revell, Kin Millen, Bill Petersen, and Linda Holland, for their vision, belief, and encouragement. A special kudo to Lela Gilbert whose gift of organization and editorial ability helped the manuscript flow and Lyra Heller for her herbal expertise. Finally, thanks to the God who placed within us the desire to pursue excellence, love people, and feel deeply.

Seeing the Big Picture

We have survived our teens, enjoyed our twenties, faced the challenges of our thirties, and—reluctantly or not—have moved into our forties and perhaps beyond. Now that we are here, facing the second half of our life, each of us has three possible choices to make with regard to our health.

In a way, the choices have always been there. But as we reach midlife, the importance of those choices becomes extremely significant. Menopause is not a disease, but it occurs at a time in our life when we are confronted with physical realities that force us to make changes in the way we are going to live our remaining years. If we don't make those changes at midlife, the future can become very bleak. If we do, we provide ourselves with the best possible chance for optimal living.

The choices that we face are quite simple:

1. We can ignore whatever is going on in our body and risk developing a degenerative disease that will negatively affect the way we live our life.
2. We can choose to treat the symptoms we are experiencing without looking for their source. (That, however, is a little like turning off the smoke alarm and going back to sleep.)
3. We can attack the underlying cause of our disease, treat it, then reach a place of optimal health and maintain that state of wellness.

Getting to a state of wellness is a very individual thing. Mark Percival, founder of Health Coach Systems International says, "It is generally not the disease but ignorance or neglect of the remedy that undermines the quality of one's life."[1] This is especially true in our middle years when conditions and symptoms gradually manifest themselves in our lives, and we stoically ignore them until they seem normal to us.

One of the reasons we do this is because most of us have entertained the false idea that to be healthy means that we have to give up what is fun. But it's really the opposite that is true. We can't get healthy by doing things that *aren't* fun. Good health is a combination of physical fitness, mental attitude, and spiritual well-being. It does not require eating birdseed, running daily marathons, or retiring to a convent. Good health opens us up to the fullness of life and does not diminish life through obsessive worry. We needn't concern ourselves with a list of things we think we should do, and then proceed to feel guilty about not doing them. Only those things we actually do will change our lives.

A REGIMEN AS UNIQUE AS YOU ARE

As we survey our unique body, personality, physical challenges, and environment, we have to look at what is strong, and build on what we have going for us. We all as individuals possess attributes that are working in our favor healthwise, just as we also have specific challenges.

We need to impact our well-being by building on the things we do well. For instance, some of us tolerate stress well. Some of us flourish while committed to a demanding physical exercise program. Some of us have tremendous endurance. Some of us really know how to celebrate life.

Besides reflecting on our strengths, we also can explore our present habits and ponder the contributions they make to our lives. Consider, for example, the way we eat—every meal that we eat either enhances or diminishes our health. Food is the most powerful drug we put in our body. According to a Surgeon General's report, 68 percent of all deaths are nutrition related.[2] We hear about drugs. We know about smoking. We've learned about alcohol. But many of us are killing ourselves with food.

Knowing our strengths and weaknesses is invaluable. But whatever the state of our health, or the genetic pattern we've inherited, every single one of us is capable of improving our state of wellness, even if we have a disease. Although we may suffer from serious heart disease or even cancer, we can make our state of wellness better through good nutrition, stress management, exercise, and ongoing mental and spiritual stimulation. The impact of such things can be made without cost. But the motivation has to come from within. We need to live by intention, not by accident.

What are the things that help people change? Our philosophy is people have within them the power to live better lives. There are many things we have the ability to do to make our lives better and to improve our overall well-being. Of course, different people have different levels of optimal health. I (Mary Ann) unfortunately learned this the hard way. I have had, at one time or another, everything imaginable wrong with me. The escalating deterioration of my health at midlife and my personal struggle have been great motivating factors in what Dr. Mayo and I do. It is the reason we have expanded our resources to include natural medicine.

A REAL MIDLIFE CRISIS

At thirty I had a bilateral mastectomy. Over the next few years my reconstructive surgery, which involved silicone implants, caused me a great deal of difficulty. I developed a nodule on my thyroid and was overdosed on thyroid medication. Consequently I lost calcium and bone strength. Eventually I developed Hashimoto's disease, an autoimmune form of hypothyroidism likely triggered by my body's reaction to years of exposure to leaking silicone. I began to have horrible joint pain. At one time my pain was so severe that Dr. Mayo and I built our house with a straight staircase because we assumed that I would eventually need a lift to get up the stairs. I seemed to be a likely candidate for a wheelchair.

Meanwhile, as the years increased, I experienced a worsening fatigue condition so that after being active all my life, every time

I exercised, I found myself so profoundly exhausted it took three days to recover. My lifelong battle with spondylothesis, a chronic back problem, worsened to the point that my physician announced I had an eighty-year-old back. Finally, I hit menopause early, after a lifetime of breezing through most of my periods and wondering what the PMS fuss was all about. It was a humbling experience.

For the first time I learned the profound effect hormones can have on your emotions, memory, and sense of well-being. I felt depressed for no reason and could not recall words. My increasingly fuzzy mind became convinced that I was now taking the first step on my mother's road toward the madness of Alzheimer's disease. Although my tests were normal, indicating that I wasn't menopausal, I began to take hormones. At that time, I didn't know about natural choices. Within two weeks, hormone replacement brought my mind back and restored my sense of well-being. One year later, tests indicated that I had officially dropped into the perimenopausal category, but as with other women sharing my hormonal journey, the symptoms appeared, disappeared, and reappeared.

My health rapidly deteriorated as I edged closer to fifty. Increasing aches and pains, general lethargy, and deteriorating memory made my daily life a struggle. Like other midlife women, my plate was full. I was simultaneously looking after my mother, dealing with the crises and marriages of adult children, relocating home and work, and finally, coping with the death of my mother and Dr. Mayo's father within six weeks of one another. Then came the revelation that Dr. Mayo's mother was to share the same Alzheimer's fate as mine. While much of what I was dealing with was out of my control, my health wasn't. Together, my physician husband of more than thirty years and I began a concerted effort to restore my health, one step at a time.

Spurred on by new information regarding silicone breast implants, I had them removed—essentially a second bilateral mastectomy—this time with no reconstruction. The debilitating fatigue began to lift; I never again experienced the need for a three-day recovery from a workout. Within a month, 75 percent of my joint pain disappeared. It was clear that for me silicone had acted in a toxic way within my body and that my overall health, menopausal complaints, and immunity had been compromised and complicated.

There was no unified answer among our colleagues in conventional medicine as to how I could remove the toxins from my body. Most physicians denied the connection between silicone and autoimmune responses. By now I was well aware that good health isn't just about taking Motrin for joint pain, Prozac for blues, or hormone replacement therapy for everything else that ails you. Optimal health requires working on the inside and using basic good health strategies, natural products when possible, and a good nutritional program as indispensable keys to having your body help you heal. By putting these new options to work, I profoundly changed my health. My joint pain continued to disappear. My fatigue diminished.

Of course all of my challenges were worsened by menopause. Your unique challenges will be worsened during that passage too. But I want to share with you the good things I learned about alternative health care as well as about up-to-date medical expertise. Used in combination, these two elements have made an enormous difference in my life. I will always have problems, but thanks to an approach that considers my entire health, I'm the best I can be.

PERSONAL FACTORS THAT MAKE A DIFFERENCE

Now, what about you? There are several factors that contribute to the state of your present health. They are:

genetics
disease complications
nutrition
toxic exposure
emotional pain
mental aggravation
a strong support system
personal faith

Due to combinations of these various factors, menopausal women experience a constellation of symptoms and signs that can be annoying and may even seem or feel life threatening. Keep this in mind: You will never die from symptoms, but you will die of risk factors. These risk factors escalate at menopause, the most dangerous being heart disease and osteoporosis (colon cancer and Alzheimer's disease are also affected by a shortage of estrogen). Please don't ignore your symptoms. But, more important, don't overlook your risk factors, which are affected by family history and by the known threats in western culture.

The most important thing you can realize is that *change is necessary now!* No woman can make a change if she believes the change she needs to make is so huge that it is impossible. However, most of us can manage getting through a day at a time, or even an hour at a time.

Change must come in small steps. That's why we advise you to start with your most urgent problem. Then move on. It has taken a long time to get your health into its present state. It will also take a long time for you to work your way out of it.

One other element that may really help is to find a model—somebody you can look up to. Is there another woman at midlife who has responded to this time of life in health and happiness? Use her as your inspiration. We all need encouragement and support. Most of the women I've talked to have found several other women to share the process with. This doesn't have to be formal. It will more likely be ad hoc—you share your experiences by phone or over lunch with your friends.

If we are going to make changes, we need to replace fear with courage so we can anticipate success. I think that, when it comes to menopause, women fear that there is no way they can logically decide what is best. Maybe one of your friends is thrilled with her use of hormones. Another is taking herbs, meditating, and refusing to eat meat. You don't know what to do. The key is education. Once you are well educated, you are prepared to make a wise decision, which will probably be a synthesis of several options.

Just keep a few encouraging things in mind. For one thing, this passage we call menopause won't go on forever. For another, there is no perfect way to get through it—we just have to do our best. We don't have to stay on a diet perfectly; we don't have to exercise perfectly. We simply have to institute certain changes and make them work within our lifestyle. We can take small steps. We can stay focused on living out our own uniqueness. If we are willing to make the changes, take the necessary steps, and explore new and different opportunities, this season of our life can lead us into a wonderful, healthy way of living—a lifestyle we have never experienced before.

The Menopause Manager is divided into five sections. Part 1 includes the following two chapters, which provide examples of what you can do to manage your menopause with understanding, options, and wisdom. In chapter 1, you'll learn about six other women and discover the process they went through. Then in chapter 2 you'll learn about yourself and about the opportunities for optimal health that are available to you.

Part 2 describes and discusses symptoms of menopause and what you can do about them. Many of these symptoms are difficult; two can be dangerous.

Part 3 explores three key aspects of wellness—the way we eat, the way we move, and the way we think.

Part 4 examines both botanical and medical alternatives for optimal health during and after menopause.

Part 5 takes a closer look at some symptoms, questions, and perspectives to help you manage your menopause.

PART ONE

FINDING A NEW PERSPECTIVE

Remember how your hormones began to rev up when you were going through puberty? Perhaps watching your daughter make the passage is an even clearer and less painful memory. The process by which you began to experience regular periods, develop breasts, and launch the woman you were to become was not smooth sailing. Your emotions went every which way, and your body seemed to stop, start, and shudder its way along the route.

Menopause is the reverse of that process *but with a critical difference.* Your body is shutting down its reproductive capacity and, as before, transporting you into new territory. This time, however, as the transition occurs, you possess a wealth of knowledge, experience, and perspective that were nowhere to be found at age thirteen. You may share physical discomforts and adjustments with your pubescent self but little else.

Like puberty, menopause is a time of tremendous potential and possibility. But unlike its earlier counterpart, it is also the time to reflect and redirect a lifetime of learning and experience into a lifestyle of your own design—perhaps for the first time ever.

1

What Others Have Done

THE DECISION-MAKING
PROCESS

Is hormone replacement for you? Or should botanicals be your choice? Are there lifestyle changes you should make for optimal health? What, if anything, should you do now that you are entering menopause? The decision-making process is not as chancy as throwing the proverbial dart or as inevitable as death and taxes. And it certainly is not as complex as the news headlines declare. There is a reasoned approach, a method to manage your perimenopause and menopause. Following it will help you feel comfortable with your decisions, make you more likely to stay with them, and increase your odds of attaining optimal health.

Ways to evaluate your own health risks and other considerations for mapping your choices are found in chapter 2. But for now, the stories of Lucy, Breeana, Marjorie, and a few other women will help you understand the process.

LUCY'S STORY

Lucy Mandela is an active mother of two teenagers and a ten-year-old. Recently her husband, Robert, helped her celebrate her forty-fifth birthday by taking her on a Caribbean cruise. Except for her frequent hot flashes, Lucy had a great time. However, on more than one mortifying occasion, sudden encounters with uninvited body heat were obvious enough to become the topic of discussion at the dinner table.

Actually for the past six months Lucy had been waking up at night, hot and sweaty, but she hadn't given it much thought. Until the trip she had not considered the significance of the hot flashes, recognized a pattern, or entertained any thought of them worsening. Even on the cruise, she was convinced that tropical heat, extra food, and alcohol were the culprits. Later on Lucy was shocked to discover that the hot flashes followed her home like some abandoned puppy that gave no indication of wanting to leave.

Three weeks later Lucy was in the office. "Dr. Mayo," she pleaded, "I am about ready to go out of my mind. I almost stripped down to my slip sitting in your waiting room. I feel like some maniac with a blowtorch is stalking me. I've tried deep breathing, sleeping with all the windows open—I'm freezing my family out of the house. The other night I had so many waves of hot flashes I just gave in and cried. Doctor, I don't have time or patience for this. I'm only forty-five and I have regular periods. I can't be menopausal. Something else has to be wrong."

While her hot flashes were extreme, Lucy is typical. Relief of hot flashes is the prime reason perimenopausal (perimenopause is the time—sometimes as many as five years—preceding the cessation of menstruation) and menopausal women are driven to seek help. For Lucy, the solution was not to leave the office with a prescription for hormone replacement. A lot of information needed to be gathered before any correct course of action could be decided.

ASSESSING THE FACTS

After she made her appointment, Lucy received an extensive package of assessment tools that measured her general health, as well as her risk factors for osteoporosis, heart disease, and diabetes. She brought them to her first visit. On that day, she was also asked to complete a standardized depression scale. The intensive interview that followed elicited her family's medical history, her personal philosophy, and general mental health.

Lucy then received an overview of menopause. She realized her young age and regular periods did not preclude her being perimenopausal. She learned other signs of menopause and recognized that she had been experiencing some of them. For example, at times her thinking had become decidedly fuzzy and she was having trouble remembering names of things, a problem she had dismissed as a sign of stress.

Laboratory work was ordered to evaluate her hormonal, thyroid, and lipid profiles. An appointment was made the following week for a baseline bone density test. Before leaving, Lucy watched a video and took home a package of reading material on menopause. Included was a checklist of natural interventions to deal with her hot flashes. She put them to immediate use. She was scheduled to return in two weeks.

On her second visit Lucy and Dr. Mayo were able to focus entirely on treatment. Lucy had done her homework and understood more about her options.

LUCY'S CHOICES

Basics of Good Health

In two weeks, by making a few dietary changes (adding vitamin E and flaxseed oil) and exercising more, Lucy was aware that she had some control over hot flashes. She hoped good health practices would help avoid or reduce the need for further intervention. She knew, for example, a concerted effort could make a difference in avoiding serious health concerns, such as heart disease—the incidence of which is reduced with a good diet, exercise, and reduction of fats and stress. A similar approach for menopausal symptoms made sense.

Complementary/Botanical

Lucy considered expanding her good health practices by adding complementary and/or botanical interventions. With them, her

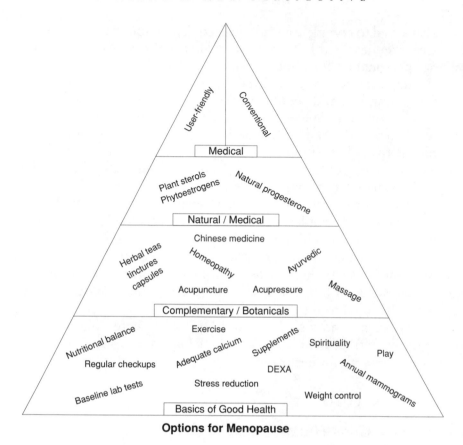

Options for Menopause

goal would be to restore health by reestablishing functional balance within her body. She would not be adding estrogen or progesterone, and no prescription would be necessary for the purchases she would make from a knowledgeable practitioner or a good nutrition or health food outlet. She could also use other natural interventions, like acupuncture or acupressure for her hot flashes. These therapies might be covered by her insurance if her physician requested them.

Natural/Medical

It's not surprising that Lucy had never heard of interventions that we refer to as natural/medical. The technology that enables plant estrogens and progesterones—changed into a form the body can use—to be bioactive and bioavailable is relatively new. These "quasi-medicines," as leading naturopathic physician Tori Hudson calls them, are considered "stronger than a botanical but weaker than a medicine."[1] The amount of estrogen and progesterone they supply is much less than medical hormone replacement. There is no question that natural/medical interventions relieve symptoms, and research is beginning to demonstrate how effectively such choices protect women against cardiovascular and osteoporotic risk.

To date, natural progesterone in combination with medically prescribed estrogen have proven to be the most effective combination in raising HDL and lowering LDL and cholesterol. Other ongoing studies suggest additional positive outcomes.

Conventional Medicine

Conventional medical intervention for menopause relieves symptoms by replacing estrogen and progestogens. Ample proof exists of this treatment's protective properties for lowering the incidence of heart disease and osteoporosis. And there is ever-increasing evidence that it decreases the risk and reduces symptoms of Alzheimer's disease and colon cancer.

Estrogen replacement therapy (ERT) or hormone replacement therapy (HRT) must be obtained by prescription. "User-friendly" medical intervention, a term first used by Tori Hudson, N.D., differs from synthetic hormone replacement because the source of the hormone is either the wild yam or soy, and the hormone replaces estrone, the form of estrogen most commonly found in menopausal women. Combined with micronized natural progesterone, some women consider it a "gentler" intervention that still guarantees protection against heart disease and osteoporosis and other estrogen-related disorders. The use of this "weaker" form of estrogen rather than estradiol—the most potent and common form of estrogen in younger women—may require some women to be particularly conscientious about maximizing good health practices in order to obtain the level of symptom relief they seek.

29

LUCY'S RISK FACTORS

An evaluation of Lucy's risk factors obtained from her history and the assessment instruments indicated low risk for heart disease, osteoporosis, diabetes, colon cancer, and Alzheimer's. Laboratory test results confirmed good lipid profiles (which measure the cholesterol level, LDL/HDL ratio, and triglycerides) and the DEXA (dual-energy X-ray absorptiometry, which measures bone density) results placed her in an appropriate range for her age. Her FSH (follicle-stimulating hormone) level (45) indicated she was indeed entering the menopause. Lucy was surprised when she talked to her mother and discovered she had become menopausal at age forty. All in all, Lucy's health risks—those that could be affected by changes in estrogen levels—were confirmed to be low.

Lucy's Rating of Her Perimenopause and Menopause Risk Factors

Risk	Good Health Principles	Low Risk	Moderate Risk	High Risk
Osteoporosis	exercise, calcium, magnesium	X		
Cardiovascular	exercise, nutrition, vitamin E, weight control, stress control, aspirin, ginkgo	X		
Alzheimer's disease	ginkgo, vitamin E, B-complex, folic acid, B12	X		
Colon cancer	nutrition, aspirin, friendly flora/probiotics	X		
Diabetes	nutrition, weight control	X		

Treatment Options:
Low to moderate risk—complementary/botanical or natural/medical
Moderate to high risk—medical

Lucy's Rating of Her Perimenopause and Menopause Symptoms

Symptom	Good Health Principles	Mild	Moderate	Severe
Hot flashes/ night sweats	exercise, essential oils, vitamin E			X
Sleep problems	exercise, stress reduction, lavender oil, calcium, magnesium, valerian, B6		X	

Symptom	Good Health Principles	Mild	Moderate	Severe
Fatigue	balanced life, stress reduction, exercise, balanced nutrition, B-complex			
Vaginal dryness	essential oils, vitamin E, regular sexual relations			
Urinary problems	essential oils, vitamin E, Kegel exercises			
Irregular bleeding	herbal tonics, dong quai, black cohosh, blue cohosh			
Joint/muscle pain	exercise, balanced nutrition, black cohosh, EFA			
Dry skin	essential fatty acids, vitamin E			
Headaches	exercise, stress reduction, balanced nutrition, magnesium			
Sexual/ desire changes	healthy relationships, Kegel exercises			
Anxiety	exercise, spiritual balance, stress reduction, salvia			
Anger/ irritability	exercise, stress reduction, B-complex, vitamins			
Depression/ mood swings	exercise, stress reduction, spiritual balance, Saint-John's-wort, B-complex			
Memory/ concentration	exercise, stress reduction, ginkgo, folic acid, B-complex		X	
Cravings	balanced nutrition, stress reduction, B-complex, vitamins			

Other:

Treatment Options:
Mild symptom—complementary/botanical
Mild to moderate symptom—natural/medical
Moderate to severe symptom—medical

LUCY'S DECISION
ON THE USE OF INTERVENTIONS

After considering all her options, and armed with the knowledge that her risk factors were low, Lucy decided to control her hot flashes with limited intervention. The suggestions she had already begun incorporating had helped, but the flashes were still a major nightly problem. She and Dr. Mayo determined that cimicifuga extract, a well-researched botanical, would be a starting point, along with a series of acupuncture treatments. For her mental fogginess and forgetfulness, she was advised to take ginkgo. For the first time in her life she began to take daily vitamins and calcium supplements.

Lucy understood that she might receive more immediate and complete relief by taking hormone replacement. But, at least in the beginning, she preferred not using "such a big gun," if she could manage her hot flashes in other ways. For the present the multiple interventions were adequate. In the future, if menopausal symptoms and/or risks changed, a new regime might be in order. In the meantime she is keeping a menopausal diary of symptoms.

Lucy kept a record of her risk factors and baseline tests that will be gauges for future decisions. Most important, she feels confident her decisions are based on an accurate understanding of her current state of health and knowledge of available options. The process of decision making brought greater clarity and understanding to the changes and adjustments she was facing—she felt prepared for the journey. The increased sensitivity to her own body maximizes her chance of achieving optimal health.

Here is a summary of how Lucy determined her correct menopausal course:

1. She gathered information.
2. She took stock of her own general health, health practices, and philosophy.
3. She educated herself about her options.

Lucy's Menopause Diary

On a scale of 1–3 keep track of your menopausal symptoms: 1=mild 2=moderate 3=severe

Day of the Month

Symptoms	1	2	3	4	5	6	7	8	9	10	11	12	13	14	15	16	17	18	19	20	21	22	23	24	25	26	27	28	29	30	31
Hot flashes	3	3	1	1	1	3	3	3	2	1	3	2	2	1	1	1	3	3	3	2	2	2	1	2	3	3	2				
Night sweats	2	2	1	1	1	1	1	1	2	2	3	2	2	1	1	1	2	2	3	2	2	2	1	3	2	2	2				
Sleeplessness										2							2	2	2	2	2	2									
Fatigue																															
Vaginal dryness																															
Irregular bleeding																															
Urinary problems																															
Joint/muscle pain																															
Dry skin																															
Headaches																															
Sexual/desire change																															
Anxiety						1	1	1	1								1	1	1												
Anger/irritability						2	2	2																							
Depression																															
Mood swings							2	2																							
Memory/concentration	1	1	1			1	1		2	2	2			2	2	2			2	2	2										
Cravings																							1			1					
Other																															

4. She determined her health risks.
5. She charted her menopausal symptoms.
6. She determined a plan of action.
7. She kept a menopause diary.

BREEANA'S STORY

Breeana is a fifty-year-old advertising executive. When she came to the office, she had been married for five years to Tom, whom she describes as "the love of my life." She had one married daughter from a previous marriage, who had recently made her a grandmother. Breeana was thrilled with her granddaughter but stunned by the fact that she had entered a new stage of life, one that had once seemed so far off. Her world was fast paced, but then, so was Breeana.

Breeana had come into the office only because it was required. Despite her pleas, unless she had a physical checkup, her company refused to renew her life insurance.

"I'm sorry I'm late," she exclaimed, dropping her overstuffed briefcase at her feet with a thud. "Do you think I'll be very long? I'm perfectly healthy. I just need a paper saying so." Breeana reached into her briefcase and from a mass of papers extricated the assessment package she had received. She had managed to fill out most of it between meetings, at lunch, or on her evening ride home on the Sausalito ferry.

As with Lucy, a thorough history was taken, the assessments evaluated, and lab tests ordered. An appointment was made for a DEXA scan. Armed with information (she had no time to watch the video), she was scheduled for a return visit in two weeks to review her results.

On her return, having looked over the materials and taken time out to think about her health, Breeana was clearly in less of a rush. In fact she was looking forward to having some questions answered. What was causing her irregular periods? What could be done about the gnawing depression that languished just beneath the surface? Was there anything that would alleviate the vaginal dryness that had made her usually satisfying sex life miserable? In addition, as energetic as she appeared to be, keeping up her pace was no longer fun. It had become an effort. For the first time she recognized that such changes might be related to menopause.

BREEANA'S RISK FACTORS

Breeana's outgoing personality gave her the appearance of being the picture of health. Her tests and history told a different story. Her father had died of a heart attack at fifty years old. Her mother had high blood pressure. Her lipid panels and blood pressure indicated that Breeana might well be in serious trouble.

To make matters worse, her bone density results showed she was osteopenic, the first step before development of osteoporosis. She had always believed her sturdy Mediterranean stock would keep her bones strong. However, her years as a smoker and the fact she rarely exercised had taken their toll. Laboratory tests revealed that she was suffering from hypothyroidism, a probable contributor to her feelings of depression and lethargy. Her lipid panel recorded her cholesterol at 266, HDL at 30, and elevated LDL of 180 (all out of the healthy range). Her FSH level (50) clearly indicated she was menopausal.

As the actual state of her health unfolded, Breeana became concerned. Like Lucy, she had familiarized herself with her treatment options, but it was not until she and Dr. Mayo were placing her risk factors on the graph that she realized how clear her choice would be.

Breeana's Rating of Her Perimenopause and Menopause Risk Factors

Risk	Good Health Principles	Low Risk	Moderate Risk	High Risk
Osteoporosis	exercise, calcium, magnesium			X
Cardiovascular	exercise, nutrition, vitamin E, weight control, stress control, aspirin, ginkgo			X
Alzheimer's disease	ginkgo, vitamin E, B-complex, folic acid, B12	X		

(Continued)

35

Risk	Good Health Principles	Low Risk	Moderate Risk	High Risk
Colon cancer	nutrition, aspirin, friendly flora/probiotics	X		
Diabetes	nutrition, weight control	X		

Treatment Options:
  Low to moderate risk—complementary/botanical or natural/medical
  Moderate to high risk—medical

Breeana's Rating of Her Perimenopause and Menopause Symptoms

Symptom	Good Health Principles	Mild	Moderate	Severe
Hot flashes/ night sweats	exercise, essential oils, vitamin E			
Sleep problems	exercise, stress reduction, lavender oil, calcium, valerian, magnesium, B6			
Fatigue	balanced life, stress reduction, exercise, balanced nutrition, B-complex		X	
Vaginal dryness	essential oils, vitamin E, regular sexual relations		X	
Urinary problems	essential oils, vitamin E, Kegel exercises		X	
Irregular bleeding	herbal tonics, dong quai, black cohosh, blue cohosh			
Joint/muscle pain	exercise, balanced nutrition, black cohosh, EFA			
Dry skin	essential fatty acids, vitamin E			
Headaches	exercise, stress reduction, balanced nutrition, magnesium			
Sexual/ desire changes	healthy relationships, Kegel exercises		X	
Anxiety	exercise, spiritual balance, stress reduction, salvia			
Anger/ irritability	exercise, stress reduction, B-complex			

Symptom	Good Health Principles	Mild	Moderate	Severe
Depression/ mood swings	exercise, stress reduction, spiritual balance, Saint-John's-wort, B-complex			
Memory/ concentration	exercise, stress reduction, ginkgo, folic acid, B-complex		X	
Cravings	balanced nutrition, stress reduction, B-complex, vitamins			
Other:				

Treatment Options:
Mild symptom—complementary/botanical
Mild to moderate symptom—natural/medical
Moderate to severe symptom—medical

BREEANA'S DECISION

It was apparent to both Dr. Mayo and Breeana that she needed estrogen protection for both her cardiovascular and osteoporosis risks. But relying on estrogen to keep her healthy and her bones strong simply was not enough. Breeana had to change her lifestyle. She modified her eating habits and began taking supplements. Lunch was now at the gym, not Georgio's. Instead of reading the paper or filling out forms on the way to work, she used the time to pray and think positively about her day and the people she would meet. She successfully kept her stress down by practicing FREEZE FRAME techniques (see chapter 15).

Thyroid medication was prescribed for her hypothyroidism. Her hormone replacement choice, made after considerable discussion, was Premarin in combination with natural progesterone, taken cyclically because she was still having periods. Dr. Mayo advised her to take a baby aspirin every other day to further protect her heart and to be diligent about taking her vitamin E and calcium.

Much of their time was spent evaluating the wisdom of hormone replacement therapy against her high risk factor: Her older

37

sister had developed breast cancer at age fifty-eight. Breeana decided that as long as she was on HRT, she would periodically monitor her levels of estrogen through a female hormone panel. That way she could insure her hormone levels were being maintained at "replacement" levels only.

She began a health calendar and included the date for yearly mammograms. An annual mammogram from fifty years on decreases the mortality and morbidity for breast cancer by 70 percent. Her goal was to keep her immunity strong through lifestyle and dietary changes. Although Breeana could have been screened for the breast cancer gene, she decided against it for fear of losing her insurance.

You'll note that Breeana had few obvious symptoms of menopause. Yet her decision for HRT was a wise one considering her health risks. Happily, within a few weeks, her greater sense of well-being returned because of the interventions of thyroid medication, HRT, and exercise. Her only obvious symptom of menopause, vaginal dryness, was relieved by the combination of estrogen vaginal cream and oral hormones.

MARJORIE'S STORY

Marjorie was forty-eight years old. Until the last four months, her life had been moving along on a fairly even keel. Nowadays, however, she would drop into bed, exhausted from chasing two-year-olds at the day care she operated, only to find herself wide awake somewhere between 1:30 A.M. and 2:45 A.M. every night. Sometimes she would fall into a deep sleep just before her alarm buzzed the unwelcome announcement that another day had begun. Much of the time, she felt irritated and angry.

Marjorie's dream had always been to run her own business and she loved working with children. The combination of these two factors in her day-care center had been a brilliant match, so her current discontent worried her. Her body ached, her periods had become continual spotting, and on top of it all, she had lost all interest in sex.

MARJORIE'S DECISION

Not being a strong believer in conventional medicine, Marjorie had already experimented with a variety of botanical interventions. While they helped, her worsening symptoms made it clear something else was needed. She had heard about "natural" estrogens and progesterones and discussed with Dr. Mayo the possibility of giving them a try.

After assurance that her risk factors were appropriate, Dr. Mayo wrote Marjorie a prescription for Triest (10 percent estradiol, 10 percent estrone, and 80 percent estriol—the weakest of the three estrogens in the body) and micronized progesterone capsules, compounded at a local pharmacy. She was instructed to keep a menopause diary. If she wanted to avoid the need for conventional medical hormone replacement, initiating and sticking to good health habits was going to be important.

> Think about it . . . What would happen to your attitude and health choices, if you were to view symptoms of menopause as passages into a place of wisdom, maturity, insight, and peace?

As for all of Dr. Mayo's menopausal patients, a follow-up appointment was scheduled in two months. By that time Marjorie's symptoms had improved—except for one. Her sexual desire had, if anything, gotten worse. This concerned Marjorie enough to consider for the first time more conventional forms of therapy. After reviewing some of the aspects of good sexual functioning, the decision was made to see if her sexual interest would improve with Estratest, a hormone that contains both estrogen and testosterone. There was slightly less than a 50 percent chance it would help, but at her two-month recheck, Marjorie reported it had helped and, as a bonus, she was also experiencing a greater sense of well-being.

ELISIA, KAYLENE, AND GWEN

"I have never experienced anything like it. I sat in my principal's office and bawled. For one of the first times in my life I was out of control. Fortunately he was sympathetic, let me cry, and gave me permission to do whatever was necessary to feel better. I left the office and went straight to my OB-GYN's office. He started me on conventional hormone therapy and within two weeks I began to feel like my old self. I am completely pleased."

For Elisia, risk factors were secondary to her general feelings of despair and of being out of control. Fortunately her body and overall health were such that hormone replacement was a solution for the symptoms she felt she had no time for and no patience with. Her routine continues to be straightforward and trouble free.

The experience of her friend and fellow teacher Kaylene was different. She was generally uncomfortable with the idea of hormone replacement but she gave it a try because nothing else alleviated her aches, pains, high heart attack risk, and the depression that accompanied her forty-ninth birthday. But her body rebelled. Different brands and methods of treatment all left her feeling worse. After months of switching from one product to another, she stopped taking everything. Unfortunately Kaylene wasn't inclined to look into lifestyle factors and overall health issues that might hold a key to relieving her misery and heart attack risk. She has chosen instead to simply grin and bear the poor health she sees as her lot in life. She chalks all of her physical problems up to menopause.

And finally, there is Gwen. A dynamic woman nearing her sixty-fifth birthday, Gwen chose to weather the storms of menopause as naturally as possible. Despite the fact that she had high risk factors for heart disease and osteoporosis and suffered severe hot flashes, she opted to forego hormonal therapy. Her doctor insisted, but there were several women in Gwen's family who had had breast cancer and their deaths made her determined to avoid anything that might contribute to her experiencing the same fate. Unlike Kaylene, however, she chose not to simply endure. Instead, she reduced her risks and symptoms by a commitment to a lifestyle that would result in optimal health. She began to eat organically, incorporating soy products into her diet as much as possible. She did a gut detoxification program. She started taking daily walks, which eventually led her to take a group of like-minded women on long, rigorous hikes every weekend. She used natural sources to control hot flashes and a combination of Chinese botanicals to support adrenal and overall health. Her weight dropped to a healthy range and her mental outlook was excellent.

Gwen is an inspiration to her friends. Her heart attack risk is now below average and she carefully monitors her bone loss, which has slowed considerably from earlier years.

What is it that we can learn from all these women? Clearly, that there is no one correct journey for all women. The decision each individual woman makes, however, should be an informed one. Hormone replacement should be honestly considered if risk factors indicate that she might benefit from it. However, one's philosophical outlook, willingness to commit to good health practices, even monetary concerns are also elements that may appropriately influence against hormones.

One need not apologize for any decision that is made—as long as the decision has been a considered one. Most important, no matter how the menopause years affect you or the presence of other health issues you may be dealing with, there is one important truth that we all share—each one of us can improve our overall wellness.

AND WHAT ABOUT YOU?

All but one of these women actively participated in making wise decisions about their menopausal experiences. Those decisions were not based on flights of fancy, on what their friends had done, or on a doctor's sole recommendation. Their choices evolved out of an evaluation of their unique health history and the current state of their health. In addition, they gathered information, took into account financial and philosophical concerns, and considered the input from their physician. Their model is your model. Let's take a look at you—your symptoms, your risks, and your options.

2

What about You?

MAKING DECISIONS ABOUT MENOPAUSE INTERVENTIONS

We've seen the process by which Lucy, Breeana, and Marjorie made decisions about the use of hormone replacement. The conclusions they reached were personal, educated, and well-reasoned. They were based on personal risk factors and symptomology.

Their decisions must be regularly reevaluated, modified, or completely altered, depending on changing risk patterns, hormonal fluctuations, and menopausal status.

Now, let's consider you and your unique situation. Should you consider hormone replacement therapy or other menopausal interventions? If so, what kind? To find out, use the same tools that Lucy, Breeana, Marjorie, and the others did. *The Menopause Manager* will help you:

gather information
evaluate your health
understand the options
determine risk
chart risk
develop an action plan

STEP ONE: GATHER INFORMATION

There are five components to gathering information:

1. education
2. your medical history
3. family history
4. lifestyle
5. laboratory results

Education

Part 1 of *The Menopause Manager* summarizes the most common signs of menopause. Other books are available that take a more anecdotal and psychosocial look at midlife, and you may want to explore them too. Read, talk to your friends, and gain a broad perspective of what menopause means to you physically, emotionally, and socially. Your goal is to develop choices that will maximize your midlife health.

Medical/Family/Lifestyle History

Health problems that look like menopause or that make menopause symptoms worse include thyroid disease, PMS, stress, intestinal/toxic effects, adrenal burnout, smoking, lack of exercise, alcohol abuse, and depression. These concerns must be assessed and attended to so that maximum relief is obtained from any menopausal intervention. Adequate evaluation and history ensure that treatment is properly focused. Our practice of looking at all these health issues is one of the major differences between what we do and how menopause is traditionally approached.

Your medical history is valuable but it is not complete without knowing the health issues of your family of origin. If you haven't done so, talk to your mother, aunts, or other surviving family members to gain information about breast cancer, heart disease, or any other relevant conditions that may have affected women in your family.

Laboratory Results

This period of time, just as you are entering the perimenopause or menopause, is a prime opportunity for you to gather baseline health information. This information will provide a standard by which you can judge how changing hormone patterns are impacting your health in the years to come.

There are twelve different tests that may be needed to establish your health baselines. Here are some general guidelines to follow:

1. Lipid profile (heart health)
   How often: If normal, every 4–5 years
   Results: Cholesterol—200 or below is good; 240 is high
   HDL—for women, below 50 is considered bad
   LDL—below 130 is good; above 160 is bad
   Triglycerides—above 190 milligrams per deciliter (mg/dl) is considered high
2. Blood chemistry panel (measures many body chemistries)
   How often: If normal, every 4–5 years; every year after age 65
   Results: There are many different panels and the results are compared to normal values
3. Hemoglobin A1C (diabetes)
   How often: At age 45 and as symptoms (thirst, hunger, frequent urination) dictate or with family history
   Results: Normal range 4.7–6.4; estimated mean blood glucose 70–110 mg/dl (if fasting glucose test is used, below 125 mg/dl)
4. Bone density test
   How often: Baseline between ages 40 and 45, then every 1–2 years depending on findings
   Results: Compared to women your age and healthy young adult women (30 years old)
5. Mammogram
   How often: Every year after age 40; baseline at age 35 with a family history of breast cancer
   Results: Interpreted by a radiologist

6. Female hormone panel
   How often: As needed for diagnosis of menopause
   Results: FSH (follicle-stimulating hormone)—above 40
   means you are menopausal; signs can begin at 20
   Perimenopausal women—preovulatory range (milli international units per milliliter—MIU/ml) 1.5–11.4; ovu-
   latory range 5.1–34.2; postovulatory range 1.1–8.4;
   compared to postmenopause of 27.6–132.9
   Female hormone panel—used to monitor hormone therapy, baseline hormone levels, and to determine the type
   and dosage of hormones needed
7. Thyroid
   How often: Baseline at 40–45 years or when symptomatic
   Results: TSH (thyroid-stimulating hormone)—normal
   range of .75–5.5
8. Adrenal stress, gut permeability, DHEA blood level
   How often: As indicated by history and symptoms
   Results: Adrenal—24-hour cortisol levels, compared to a
   normal range
   DHEA level—350–2,000 micrograms per deciliter (mcg/dl)
   in women
   Gut/liver—measures abnormal gut permeability/liver
   toxicity
9. Blood pressure
   How often: Every 1–2 years, if normal
   Results: Persistent high blood pressure is significant; a
   few sporadic high blood pressure measurements are
   not
10. Pap test
    How often: Annually beginning at age 18; earlier if sexu-
    ally active; more often with abnormal findings such as
    atypia or dysplasia
    Results: Report by a pathologist
11. Colorectal cancer screening
    How often: Fecal occult blood test—annually after 50;
    sigmoidoscopy—every 5 years
    Results: Interpreted by a professional

12. Colposcopy and biopsy
    How often: Following a pap test if atypia or dysplasia persists or progresses in severity
    Results: Report by a pathologist
13. Endometrial biopsy
    How often: When there is persistent erratic bleeding
    Results: Report by a pathologist

We recommend five exams that should be done on a regular basis. Here are general guidelines for each:

1. Breast exam
   How often: Monthly self-exam; once a year by a physician, especially after age 40
   Results: Lumps may require nonsurgical or surgical follow-up
2. Gynecological exam
   How often: Yearly or as advised or when there is a concern; anytime you have unexplained bleeding after menopause
   Results: Follow-up as advised by your physician
3. Skin exam
   How often: Self-exam every 3 months; anytime there are changes in existing warts, moles, freckles, or there are new growths
   Results: Follow-up as advised by your physician
4. Eye exam
   How often: If no symptoms, every 2–4 years between ages 40 and 64; every 1–2 years if 65 or older
   Results: Follow-up as advised by your physician
5. Dental exam
   How often: Two times a year
   Results: Follow-up as advised by your dentist

STEP TWO: EVALUATE THE STATE OF YOUR HEALTH

At A Woman's Place we use a variety of assessment tools developed to evaluate functional health of the gut and liver, as well as psychological health. We use a questionnaire of nearly seven hundred questions. For your purpose, the following scale will be helpful in evaluating your overall health.

On a scale of 1–5, with 1 being optimal health, ask yourself, how am I doing?

1. My digestive system is functioning well. I have little excess gas and few episodes of constipation or diarrhea. My score:
2. I sleep soundly through the night. My score:
3. My weight is right where it should be. My score:
4. I am eating regular, well-balanced meals. My score:
5. I exercise at least 30 minutes, 3 times a week. My score:
6. Most of the time I am able to keep stress down to a reasonable level. My score:
7. I limit my caffeine to two sources a day. My score:
8. I do not drink more than one alcoholic beverage a day. My score:
9. I do not smoke. My score:

Think about it . . . The Centers for Disease Control and Prevention in their 1997 data report an increasing trend toward heterosexual transmission of HIV. If you or your partner have not had one lifelong, monogamous partner, you may be at risk.

Scores of three or more indicate an area that you need to focus on to improve your overall health. Talk over areas of concern with your doctor or consider making the changes you know are necessary.

STEP THREE: UNDERSTAND YOUR OPTIONS

The options for dealing with menopause symptoms are covered in detail in the chapters that follow. They are summarized in the chart on the following page.

47

A Woman's Place Menopause Diary

On a scale of 1–3 keep track of your menopausal symptoms: 1=mild 2=moderate 3=severe

Symptoms

Day of the Month

Symptoms	1	2	3	4	5	6	7	8	9	10	11	12	13	14	15	16	17	18	19	20	21	22	23	24	25	26	27	28	29	30	31
Hot flashes																															
Night sweats																															
Sleeplessness																															
Fatigue																															
Vaginal dryness																															
Irregular bleeding																															
Urinary problems																															
Joint/muscle pain																															
Dry skin																															
Headaches																															
Sexual/desire change																															
Anxiety																															
Anger/irritability																															
Depression																															
Mood swings																															
Memory/concentration																															
Cravings																															
Other																															

Summary of the Options for Menopause

Level One: Basics of Good Health

Whether or not you are experiencing signs of menopause, midlife is the time to reevaluate your health

Regular checkups, balanced diet, more soy, nutritional supplements, exercise, baseline laboratory tests, stress reduction, weight management, flaxseed oil, calcium, spiritual development, play

Level Two: Complementary/Botanical

Improved function and symptom relief, without adding estrogen and/or progesterone

Herbs as teas, tinctures, and capsules; massage, Ayurvedic and Chinese medicine, homeopathy, acupuncture/acupressure

Level Three: Natural/Medical

"Stronger than a botanical, weaker than a medicine." Adds weak forms of estrogen and progesterone to relieve symptoms, but limited proof as yet of cardiovascular or osteoporotic protection

Phytoestrogens and natural progesterone from plant phytosterols made bioavailable as creams, lozenges, capsules, oils, DHEA, melatonin, pregnenolone

Level Four: Medical

Adds estrogen and progestin to relieve symptoms and protect against heart disease and osteoporosis

User-friendly medical hormones are estrone, derived from the wild yam or soy; Premarin, a conjugated estrogen derived from equine urine; conventional hormones, synthesized in the laboratory

STEP FOUR: DETERMINE YOUR RISK FACTORS

The following sets of questions will help you determine if you are at risk for osteoporosis, cardiovascular disease, colon cancer, Alzheimer's disease, diabetes, and breast cancer.

Osteoporosis Risk

I have a small, thin frame or am Caucasian or Asian.	___Yes ___No
I have a family history of osteoporosis.	___Yes ___No
I am postmenopausal.	___Yes ___No
I had an early or surgically induced menopause.	___Yes ___No
I have been taking excessive thyroid medication or high doses of cortisone-based drugs (steroids) for asthma, arthritis, or cancer.	___Yes ___No
I am physically inactive.	___Yes ___No
I smoke cigarettes or have a high alcohol intake (more than 4 oz. a day).	___Yes ___No

Add the yes answers for your score. A score of 4 or more is high, 2–3 is moderate, and 0 or 1 is low.
My osteoporosis risk is ___Low ___Moderate ___High

Cardiovascular Risk

I have a mother, sister, or daughter who had a heart attack, stroke, or coronary bypass before age 65.	___Yes ___No
I have a father, brother, or son who had a heart attack, stroke, or coronary bypass before age 55.	___Yes ___No
I have a high alcohol intake and/or smoke.	___Yes ___No

I have diabetes.	___Yes ___No
My triglycerides are over 200.	___Yes ___No
My lipid profile is abnormal.	___Yes ___No
I am physically inactive.	___Yes ___No
I am under high stress.	___Yes ___No
I am overweight and carry my weight mostly around my middle.	___Yes ___No
I eat a high-fat diet and lots of red meat.	___Yes ___No

Add the yes answers for your score. If you answered yes to statements 1 or 2 or if you have 5 or more yes answers, your score is high, 3–4 is moderate, and 0–2 is low.

My cardiovascular disease risk is ___Low ___Moderate ___High

Colon Cancer Risk

I have a close relative with colon cancer.	___Yes ___No
I am experiencing rectal bleeding and/or changes in bowel habits and stool appearance, especially rectal bleeding.	___Yes ___No
I eat a high-fat diet, low in fiber.	___Yes ___No

Add the yes answers for your score. A yes to statement 1 counts as 2 points. A score of 3 or more is high, 2 is moderate, and 0–1 is low.

My colon cancer risk is ___Low ___Moderate ___High

Alzheimer's Risk

I have a mother or father with Alzheimer's disease or "dementia."	___Yes ___No
I have several relatives with Alzheimer's disease or "dementia."	___Yes ___No

Add the yes answers. A score of 2 is high, 1 is moderate, 0 is low.

My Alzheimer's disease risk is ___Low ___Moderate ___High

Diabetes Risk

Diabetes runs in my family.	___Yes	___No
I am overweight.	___Yes	___No
I was diabetic when I was pregnant.	___Yes	___No
I carry my extra weight around my middle.	___Yes	___No
I do not eat well.	___Yes	___No

Add the yes answers. A score of 4 or more is high, 2–3 is moderate, 0–1 is low.

My diabetes risk is ___Low ___Moderate ___High

Breast Cancer Risk

I have the breast cancer (BRCA1 and/or BRCA2) genes or family history of breast cancer. There is a 5–10 percent chance of carrying the BRCA1 gene.	___Yes	___No
I get limited exercise.	___Yes	___No
I started my periods before age 12.	___Yes	___No
I had a late menopause, after age 51.	___Yes	___No
I am childless or had my first child after age 35.	___Yes	___No
I eat a high-fat diet with limited vegetables.	___Yes	___No
I have never breast-fed a child.	___Yes	___No
I am overweight.	___Yes	___No

Score 3 for a yes answer to statement 1. Add to the other yes answers. A score of 5 or more is high, 2–4 is moderate, 0–1 is low.

My breast cancer risk is ___Low ___Moderate ___High

STEP FIVE: CHARTING YOUR RISKS AND SYMPTOMS

Use the following charts to rate your menopause risk factors and symptoms.

Rating Your Perimenopause and Menopause Risk Factors

Risk	Good Health Principles	Low Risk	Moderate Risk	High Risk
Osteoporosis	exercise, calcium, magnesium			
Cardiovascular	exercise, nutrition, vitamin E, weight control, stress control, aspirin, ginkgo			
Colon cancer	nutrition, aspirin, friendly flora/probiotics			
Alzheimer's disease	ginkgo, vitamin E, B-complex, folic acid, B12			
Diabetes	nutrition, weight control			

Treatment Options:
Low to moderate risk—complementary/botanical or natural/medical
Moderate to high risk—medical

Rating Your Perimenopause and Menopause Symptoms

Symptom	Good Health Principles	Mild	Moderate	Severe
Hot flashes/ night sweats	exercise, essential oils, vitamin E			
Sleep problems	exercise, stress reduction, lavender oil, calcium, magnesium, valerian, B6			
Fatigue	balanced life, stress reduction, exercise, balanced nutrition, B-complex			
Vaginal dryness	essential oils, vitamin E, regular sexual relations			
Urinary problems	essential oils, vitamin E, Kegel exercises			
Irregular bleeding	herbal tonics, dong quai, black cohosh, blue cohosh			

(Continued)

Symptom	Good Health Principles	Mild	Moderate	Severe
Joint/muscle pain	exercise, balanced nutrition, black cohosh, EFA			
Dry skin	essential fatty acids, vitamin E			
Headaches	exercise, stress reduction, balanced nutrition, magnesium			
Sexual/desire changes	healthy relationships, Kegel exercises			
Anxiety	exercise, spiritual balance, stress reduction, salvia			
Anger/irritability	exercise, stress reduction, B-complex, vitamins			
Depression/ mood swings	exercise, stress reduction, spiritual balance, Saint-John's-wort, B-complex			
Memory/ concentration	exercise, stress reduction, ginkgo, folic acid, B-complex			
Cravings	balanced nutrition, stress reduction, B-complex, vitamins			
Other:				

Treatment Options:
Mild symptom—complementary/botanical
Mild to moderate symptom—natural/medical
Moderate to severe symptom—medical

STEP SIX: A PLAN OF ACTION

Having calculated your health risks and symptoms and recorded them on the chart, you should perceive the level of intervention that may be needed to insure your good health. However, before you do anything, ask yourself the following questions.

1. Am I motivated by a desire to achieve my optimal health? If not, what is motivating me to make changes in my health or to maintain the status quo?

2. Am I willing to participate on a regular basis with my health care provider to insure that the changes I make are beneficial?

3. Am I willing to continue with whatever interventions I choose for a reasonable period of time?

4. If I am going to use natural interventions, am I choosing them because they are appropriate for my level of risk and symptomology or because I philosophically prefer them?

5. Am I willing to do my homework, read, and make sure any complementary and botanical interventions are pure, standardized products from reputable sources?

6. Am I willing to be as discerning and demanding with complementary, botanical, and other "natural" interventions as I am with conventional medical interventions?

7. Am I willing to incur the additional expense and time that may be called on for any intervention?

8. Are the decisions I have made in line with personal philosophy or, if not, am I willing to continue to develop a plan for which I have a comfortable ownership?

9. My number one health concern in the next six months is

_____.

To that end, I will _____

_____.

10. My plan for menopausal intervention, based on the information I presently have and my current state of health, is to

_____.

Record Keeping

After deciding on your plan of action, it will be important to keep good records of all tests or medications so that you can continue to make wise decisions concerning your health care. Use the following as a guide to the information you will want to keep up to date.

1. Every year in _____ I will schedule an annual checkup to reevaluate the status of my health and medical and alternative interventions.
2. Doctor's name:
   Address:
   Phone:
3. A list of allergies
4. History of hospitalizations and operations
5. List of medications:
   Medicine
   Condition
   Dose/schedule
   Date started
   Date finished
6. List of tests

Test	Date	Result
DEXA		
Blood pressure		
Total cholesterol		
Triglycerides		
HDL		
LDL		
Mammogram		
Pap		
TSH		
FSH		
Hemoglobin A1C		
Blood chemistry		
VAP (Vertical Auto Profile)		
High Sensitivity C-reactive Protein		
Homocysteine		
Ratio of two-hour post prandail glucose and insulin		

PART TWO

DISCOVERING
YOUR BODY'S
UNIQUENESS

The order in which menopausal signs and symptoms appear varies enormously. The whole menopausal process is a transition into a stage where childbearing is not the primary function of the reproductive system. Therefore, irregularities in the length of the menstrual cycle, changes in bleeding patterns, and missed periods are often among the first signs of change.

Occasional hot flashes are another early sign.

Joint pain and fatigue are appearing more frequently and earlier than they were reported in the past.

Sleep, mood, and memory disturbances often occur next.

These changes may be followed by vaginal dryness, painful coitus, urinary urgency, or incontinence.

A multitude of other signs may come and go.

The "silent" risks of menopause—heart disease and osteoporosis—manifest themselves late in the transition.

I have introduced these symptoms in their most typical order. However, your pattern may be quite different. In part 2 of *The Menopause Manager,* we'll take an in-depth look at the signs and symptoms of menopause. For each symptom, we'll discuss:

- What is happening physiologically
- Interventions that provide relief and/or protection
- How suggested interventions work and what they do

The merits and details of how, when, and what to use of natural and synthetic hormone replacement, as well as greater detail on botanical interventions, will be covered extensively in part 4. The areas you may need to address to ensure that the intervention you choose is effective and maximally utilized will be found in chapter 20.

3

Bleeding Irregularities

In midlife some women genuinely mourn the inability to become pregnant. However, with teenagers in the home or the first grandchild toddling around the living room, most of us welcome the freedom from birth control and monthly periods. In fact if this were the only change triggered by menopause, it would probably be relabeled the "pause that refreshes." Unfortunately there are other changes, and the changes in hormone balance brought on by menopause can be far-reaching and can negatively impact a woman's quality of life.

JANINE'S STORY

At forty-seven Janine's quality of life was less than enjoyable. She still remembers her fitful start into her menopausal journey. It took precedence over the trip she and her husband had planned for months. First of all, Janine began an erratic bleeding episode that rendered foreign travel less than fun. To make matters worse, she couldn't sleep and she felt depressed. Worst of all, sex was the last thing on her mind, even though this was her long-anticipated "second" honeymoon. In short, Janine could hardly wait to get home. But unfortunately her maladies did not remain on foreign shores but took on new rancor in familiar territory.

After Janine's doctor assured her she wasn't menopausal, her anxiety increased to the point where she had to listen to relaxation tapes just to get to work. One day she couldn't remember her mother's maiden name, the birthdate of her first child, or whether she had already been to the grocery store—she concluded she had Alzheimer's disease. The neurologist she consulted assured her she was fine and offered no other explanation for her symptoms. Her short-term memory and confusion increased, as did her depression. Noting her mood, a psychiatrist put her on an antidepressant, which was of minimal help.

Janine's husband insisted she see a different OB-GYN. This time she was told she *was* menopausal and needed a D & C (dilatation and curettage) to control the bleeding, but she would not be ready for hormones until she started having hot flashes. By this time Janine was fifty and at her wits' end. Frustrated with the prospect of dealing with a new physician, she anticipated her next step—a nervous breakdown, squeezed in between bleeding irregularities, and finally the long-awaited hot flashes! Janine had longed for hormones but once she began to take them, they accentuated her bleeding and she became bloated. It took several months before she and her physician found a hormonal combination that worked.

For the curious . . . According to a North American Menopause Society study, only half of working women of menopausal age were able to name health risks associated with menopause—27 percent mentioned osteoporosis; only 6 percent associated menopause with heart disease, the leading killer of women in menopause.

Janine's menopausal junket was a wild one because the directions she was given along the way were for someone else's journey.

WHAT'S HAPPENING TO MY BODY?

At the end of the menstrual process, a woman's body no longer contains eggs, thus the hormones estrogen and progesterone are no longer produced in sufficient amounts to support implantation and growth of a baby. A new chapter begins in which each woman's role moves from the bearer of a single life to a broader view—a supporter of life. In menopause, there is no longer any need for lush uterine linings. Monthly buildup of the endometrium ceases, sometimes by fits and starts, sometimes gradually, and occasionally abruptly.

Meanwhile, there may be vast differences between the symptoms that occur during the perimenopause, based on the egg that is released into the monthly cycle and the condition of that egg.

Think of it this way. Of all the ovarian follicles that have made it through approximately thirty-five years of monthly cycles, some are little worse for wear while others are clearly showing their age. An egg follicle in good shape is like a woman who has had a somewhat privileged life. She had regular medical checkups, massages, a nanny for times when her children cried, and a husband who loved her and provided a good home. Chances are she will look younger than her age and feel almost like she did when she was a teenager.

For the curious . . .
At menopause:
10 percent of women stop their periods abruptly. 18 percent experience heavier and more frequent bleeding. 70 percent find periods get lighter and irregular.[1]

An egg follicle that is degenerating is like a woman whose husband left her with three kids to care for. She smokes to "relieve" stress and she stands in the sun directing traffic six hours a day to provide food and shelter for her children. She will look older than her age, will have health problems that have been ignored, and will generally be tired and worn-out.

A month when a "well-preserved" egg follicle is stimulated will be perceived as normal, or nearly so. Any drop in hormone levels is so slight it is hardly noticeable. In contrast, a month when a "stressed" follicle is stimulated will result in unpredictable hormone levels, which cause cycle irregularities, hot flashes, and other typical signs associated with the perimenopause and menopause.

The challenge is to be able to distinguish menopausal shutdown from other less-than-healthy conditions. Menopausal shutdown causes bleeding irregularities or pattern changes that are expected and normal. However, it can resemble patterns resulting from conditions that need immediate attention, such as endometrial cancer (cancer involving the lining of the uterus), an endometrial polyp (a protruding growth), endometrial hyperplasia (overgrowth of the lining), adenomyosis (endometrial growth in the muscular portion of the uterine wall), or growth of fibroids (erratic uterine muscle growth).

WHAT CAN I DO ABOUT IRREGULAR BLEEDING?

Abnormal bleeding is bleeding that occurs erratically, at intervals of twenty-one days or less, lasts for more than seven days, is very heavy, or has a very irregular pattern.

A menstrual diary can be a great help in eliciting patterns and determining a course of action. Anemia should be ruled out and a hysteroscopic exam, D & C, and/or an endometrial biopsy can help diagnose cancer, hyperplasia, or polyps.

For the curious . . . As the follicular phase shortens, menstrual times tend to shorten from twenty-eight days to around twenty-six days by age forty.

To treat the problem nutritionally, supplement with vitamin B6, B12, and folic acid (important for proper blood cell manufacture), vitamin A and E (for healthy tissue growth), magnesium (vascular tone and smooth muscle function), and vitamin C (hormone and collagen synthesis). Don't forget your essential fatty acids (EFAs) since they are necessary for the production of prostaglandins and for a number of physiological responses like muscle contraction, vascular dilatation, and the shedding of the uterine lining.

Herbal tonics, such as chaste tree berry *(Vitex agnus-castus),* dong quai *(Angelica sinensis),* and black cohosh *(Cimicifuga racemosa),* may even out the functioning of the reproductive system, especially if symptoms are mild. Herbs known to stop bleeding include shepherd's purse *(Capsella bursa-pastoris),* agimony *(Agrimonia eupatoria),* witch hazel *(Hamamelis virginiana),* and blue cohosh *(Caulophyllum thalictroides).* Control may require the use of estrogen. After the acute episode, progesterone may be added. NSAIDS (Motrin and the like) can help, but caution is always in order since they disrupt the bowel flora and can trigger gastric discomfort (see chapter 20).

When nothing else works, surgical interventions such as a D & C or hysteroscopy (using an optical instrument to view inside the uterine lining) may help. They can be both diagnostic and therapeutic. Surgically interventions are certainly a quick way to control or stop bleeding, but the underlying pathology may still remain. Laser ablation, a relatively new technique more common in Europe, effectively controls or stops bleeding in 65–75 percent of the cases, but there is concern about whether all the endometrial tissue is removed or destroyed. The laser allows for a precise delivery of heat energy to the depth needed to eliminate the endometrial lining. There are risks associated with this procedure, from uterine perforation to intravascular fluid overload and death, and it should be used only by an experienced physician.

A future office procedure, available in the next year or so, will involve heating a balloonlike device that fills the uterine cavity and effectively destroys the endometrium. Hysterectomy should be recommended only after all other avenues have failed.

ANY OTHER SUGGESTIONS?

Hope is on the way for women who are tired of bleeding but prefer not to have to go through frequent biopsies and other procedures. Studies done on the effectiveness of using vaginal sonography (ultrasound) suggest more invasive techniques can be avoided while improving the odds of detecting serious problems.[2] Ultrasound can help the physician determine whom he or she can continue to observe, thus sparing the expense and trauma of biopsy, hysteroscopy, or other surgical intervention.

It is estimated that more than half of the women who have biopsies would be spared if they had ultrasonography first. The practice of subjecting women to a biopsy based on less than an eight-millimeter thickening of the endometrial lining, as shown with ultrasonography, when she has no symptoms and was not on hormones may be far more intervention than is called for.[3]

Women receiving hormones, who have persistent bleeding, have a higher risk of endometrial cancer and, therefore, need further testing and follow-up.

Pearls of wisdom about bleeding irregularities . . .

1. Bleeding that cannot be controlled by medical treatment may indicate cancer.
2. Diagnosis of the cause of erratic bleeding can be made a number of ways.
3. At menopause, always take erratic bleeding seriously.

Hot Flashes

Reframing how we view life's challenges helps us overcome adversity. The classic reframe for menopause is reflected in the joke, "I'm not having a hot flash—it's a power surge!" Another is the menopause support organization called The Red Hot Mamas. Nowhere is the ability to laugh and to reframe more important than with hot flashes.

During the menopause, 80 percent of all women in the United States report having hot flashes/flushes at least occasionally. The patterns vary. Some women have them years before they experience any change in their period. Others may experience their first flash after they have ceased their menses.

Many women don't associate a mild sweep of heat or getting overheated at night (night sweat) as a true hot flash. We tend to associate hot flash with the picture of a woman pouring ice down her blouse, tearing off her clothes, turning purple, or running outside. For years this consistent manifestation was the only symptom, outside cessation of periods, the medical community attributed to menopause.

WHAT IS A HOT FLASH?

To date, no one knows for sure what causes such rapid fluctuations in body temperature but there is speculation it is caused by a change in the body's core set-point that triggers dilation of surface blood vessels. Physiologically, surface blood vessels dilate, the heart beats slightly faster, and sweating occurs. Blood flows to the surface causing as much as a two-degree difference in the temperature of the skin.

While many women are occasionally mildly bothered by these episodes, others complain of inability to sleep, profuse sweating, increased heartbeat (experienced at times as palpitations), emotional exhaustion, and a generally severe interruption of their lives. The experience may even include a brief sensation of suffocation or inability to breathe and a sensation of heat rising from within and spreading upward from the chest to the neck and face.

For the curious . . . Technically a hot flash is thought to be a disorder of heat regulation triggered within the hypothalamus by norepinephrine.

The hot flash itself may be very brief, typically lasting three to six minutes, but it can last for more than thirty minutes or may be followed by waves of flashes. The length of time a woman will have hot flashes varies. Some women suffer for years and others for only a few months. Since the problem stems from temperature regulation irregularities, cold flashes are also possible, and rapid cooling after a hot flash can result in a chill. Besides those in menopause, persons who are pregnant, are under high stress, suffer from hyperthyroidism, drink a lot of alcohol, or have out-of-control diabetes may also experience hot flashes.

IS FLASHING ALL IN MY MIND?

Japanese and Mayan women have few hot flashes or else take little note of them. Some suggest that this proves the power of suggestion, because in our American culture, menopause is seen as a time of illness and misery. However, it is highly suggestive that diet, exercise habits, and/or other genetic or cultural differences play a part in how frequently hot flashes are experienced. Cultures in which women have few flashes generally have diets high in phytoestrogens and get lots of exercise. In Europe, German women appear to suffer most, Italian women least.

In addition, it is known that reduced estrogen triggers a respiratory reaction affecting the hypothalamus and leads to dilation of the small surface blood vessels in an attempt to dissipate the heat. The fact that alterations in respiration consistently occur along with hot flashes emphasizes the reality that hot flashes involve several diverse biological systems. Therefore, controlling them can involve a number of differing approaches.

REDUCING HOT FLASHES

There is no cure for hot flashes, but there is symptom relief. A literal losing of your cool can be embarrassing, especially if it is accompanied by escalating shades of red, along with sweat doing peculiar things with your makeup. But embarrassment aside, hot flashes can be distracting and make you feel miserable.

Keeping a diary is helpful for discovering patterns and will provide insight into your unique triggers. Don't underestimate the impact taking care of the obvious can have. Keep your rooms cool and avoid hot environments. Use absorbent fabrics and sheets. Avoid confining or heavy clothing or covers, hot drinks, alcohol, caffeine, chocolate, soft drinks, sugar, and spicy foods. Soothing hot baths, hot tubs, or saunas before bedtime may need to be discontinued for a while. Smoking contributes to hot flashes. And most women are well aware of the connection between stress and flashes.

For the curious . . . Twenty-five percent of women who have hot flashes have them for longer than five years.

Since vegetarians have fewer flashes, it makes sense to take their lead and cut back on animal fats and red meat and eat more vegetables. Modification of your lifestyle may be enough to see you through. If not, adding one or more of the following remedies may work. Finally, keep in mind that as unsettling as hot flashes can be, they are not life threatening, nor are they the definitive indication that you need hormone replacement.

TWENTY-ONE THINGS TO DO FOR HOT FLASHES

Try Supplements
1. vitamin E
2. vitamin C
3. bioflavonoids
4. B-complex

Try Botanicals
5. herbal teas
6. herbs

Try Specialized Herbs
7. extract of black cohosh
8. combination botanicals and vitamins

Try Homeopathy
9. homeopathic remedies

Try Dietary Additions
10. foods high in phytosterols
11. "superfoods"
12. bee pollen and royal jelly
13 essential fatty acids

Try Stress Relief
14. mental/physical relaxation

Try Physical Therapy
15. acupuncture
16. exercise

Try Natural/Medical and Medical Therapy
17. phytoestrogens and natural progesterone
18. estrogen/progestin
19. Clonidine and Megace

When All Else Fails Try
20. deep diaphragmatic breathing
21. acupressure

Try Supplements

Descriptions and details of the following supplements are found in chapter 13. Please refer to that chapter before using them.

Start your supplements with vitamin E, taking 400–800 international units (IU) daily. Increase the dosage over a two-week period and then reduce it to the lowest effective dose as your hot flashes subside. Do not go above 1,200 IU of vitamin E. If you have high blood pressure, diabetes, bleeding disorders, or rheumatic heart disease or take digitalis, consult your physician first.

Increase your vitamin C intake up to 1,000 milligrams daily. If regular ascorbic acid upsets your stomach, try a buffered brand. Vitamin C aids vitamin E absorption. An equal amount of the bioflavonoid hesperidin (1,000 milligrams in divided doses) along with vitamin C maximizes the effectiveness of vitamin C, improving vascular integrity and capillary function.

Other bioflavonoids, such as rutin and quercetin, may be helpful as well. Take 250 milligrams up to five or six times per day. Better yet, eat good, fresh foods that contain all such micronutrients: fennel, celery, parsley, flaxseed oil, nuts, seeds, lemons, grapefruit, rosehips, and buckwheat. The edible part of the fruit contains ten times more flavonoids than the juice.

Twenty-five to 100 milligrams per day of B-complex can increase vitamin E's effectiveness. Vitamin B5 (pantothenic acid) improves adrenal function. Since estrogen tends to deplete B6 (pyridoxine), supplementation is needed especially during estrogen therapy. B vitamins help reduce stress and are vital for many chemical processes.

Try Botanicals

Descriptions and details of many of the following herbals and how to ensure their effectiveness and purity are in chapter 16. Please refer to that chapter before using them.

Products containing all or some of the following herbs have been associated with women's health and may be helpful, over time, in preventing hot flashes or reducing their frequency or severity. Some herbs should not be used while you are bleeding and many are dangerous if there is any chance of pregnancy. In many cases the basis of their effectiveness on women's health is the ability of the plant phytosterols to act like estrogen or progesterone in the body. Their action, however, is only 2 percent as strong as the estrogen you make in your body.[1] Other herbs help relieve menopause symptoms by improving the body's overall functioning.

"Women's" teas are readily available. Those containing various combinations of sage, chamomile, Siberian ginseng, dong quai, fennel, black cohosh, licorice, and sarsaparilla are traditionally used to reduce hot flashes. Products containing all or some of the following herbs are likely to help with hot flashes as well as other menopausal symptoms.

Chinese/Indian Combinations	European/ North American Combinations
Dong quai root	Black cohosh root
(Angelica sinensis)	(Cimicifuga racemosa)
Rehmannia root	Wild yam
(Rehmannia glutinosa)	(Dioscorea villosa)
Codonopsis root	Hops
(Codonopsis pilosula)	(Humulus lupulus)
Ginseng root	Chaste tree berry
(Panax ginseng)	(Vitex agnus-castus)
Poria fungus	Fennel seed
(Poria cocos)	(Foeniculum vulgare)
Peony root	Anise seed
(Paeonia lactiflora)	(Pimpinella anisum)
Red sage root	Valerian root
(Salvia officinalis)	(Valeriana officinalis)
Licorice root	Motherwort herb
(Glycyrrhiza glabra)	(Leonurus cardiaca)
Ginger rhizome	Licorice root
(Zingiber officinale)	(Glycyrrhiza glabra)
Ginkgo	False unicorn root
(Ginkgo biloba)	(Chamaelirium luteum)
Siberian ginseng	Black haw
(Eleutherocoscus senticosus)	(Viburnum prunifolium)
	Cramp bark
	(Viburnum opulus)
	Lemon balm
	(Melissa officinalis)
	Saint-John's-wort
	(Hypericum perforatum)

Fem Herbal (Metagenics) and Eight Treasures (Ethical Nutrients) are classic combinations of Chinese herbal extracts in small pellets that make individualizing the dose very easy. FemTone (PhytoPharmica) is an herbal combination in a capsule.

Try Specialized Herbs

Black cohosh extract *(Cimicifuga racemosa)* is mentioned separately because, unlike many botanicals, good research has verified its usefulness in preventing hot flashes and sweating, as well as relieving nervousness, achiness, and depressive moods caused by lowered hormone levels.[2] It works on the hypothalamus, pituitary gland, and estrogen receptors.

70

Black cohosh extract is commonly used in both Germany and Australia. Its usefulness for relieving hot flashes has been known in Europe since the eighteenth century. Although it has been known by Native Americans as "rattle weed," its use has only recently increased in the United States.

At A Woman's Place we have also found particular success with products that combine vitamins that are especially vital for menopausal women, such as E, C, D, B5, B6, calcium, bioflavonoids, and PABA (para-aminobenzoic acid, which plays a role in B vitamin metabolism), and selected botanicals considered to be hormone regulators and/or supportive of the nervous system. We recommend Fem EstroPlex (Metagenics). Similar combinations can be found in health food stores by Ethical Nutrients, Enzymatic Therapy, or Zand. These products, as well as the all-herbal variety, can be taken along with hormone replacement for additional support or while transitioning on or off hormone therapy.

Try Homeopathy

The Greek words *homeos,* meaning "similar," and *pathos,* meaning "disease," sum up the approach of this system of medicine. The fundamental principle is that "like cures like." Homeopathy treats illness with dilute, but "potentised," plant, mineral, and chemical substances.

Homeopathic remedies can be purchased over the counter or prepared for the individual by a practitioner skilled in their use. A typical homeopathic formula is in liquid form or in easily dissolved tablets that are placed under the tongue for quick absorption. Traditional ingredients, listed with their potency, might include some or all of the following: lachesis 12x, sepia 12x, sanguinaria 12x, sulfuric acid 6x, pulsatilla 12x, lycopodium 6x.

Try Dietary Additions

Add foods high in phytosterols—"phytoestrogens." Considerable scientific evidence exists showing that soy products are helpful in reducing hot flashes and other signs of menopause. Try substituting soy milk in recipes and soups. Use herbed tofu in

71

place of sour cream. Don't overdo soybeans, uncooked cabbage, cauliflower, or kale if you suffer from hypothyroidism, for they are believed to contain certain thyroid-blocking substances. Other good choices of phytosterols are fennel, celery, parsley, nuts, seeds, apples, alfalfa, barley, red clover sprouts, and yams.

Try downing some of the "superfoods," or "green" drinks containing super blue-green algae, spirulina, and the like that are being sold in most health food stores. They help reduce flashes because of their high B-complex and they boost energy.

Bee pollen and royal jelly are filled with vitamins, amino acids, minerals, and all kinds of healthy-sounding ingredients that can be useful in preventing hot flashes—but a caution is in order. They can be contaminated with pollen or other substances that trigger allergic reactions and cause anaphylactic shock in susceptible people.[3]

Essential fatty acids, such as evening primrose oil, taken as capsules two to three times a day, alleviate hot flashes, possibly because of the gamma linolenic acid (GLA) in the oil, which influences prostaglandin production. Flaxseed oil, in capsules or one to three teaspoons fresh over vegetables, on toast or cereal, or in salads is very effective. Always use flaxseed oil unheated and keep it refrigerated. Borage oil can be taken as a capsule, tea, or tincture and contains saponins that have progesterone-like activity. These oils act as restorative agents to the adrenals. Since the body cannot make essential fatty acids, they must be included in the diet (more on essential fatty acids in chapter 13).

Try Stress Relief

Times of stress increase the incidence of hot flashes. Do what you can to relax and calm both yourself and your life (see chapter 15).

Try Physical Therapy

A visit to the acupuncturist may help your flashes and may be covered by your insurance since it is recognized as an effective treatment by the American College of Obstetricians and Gynecologists. Eight weeks of treatment with acupuncture once or twice a week for thirty minutes has been found to be helpful for at least three months after treatment is stopped.[4]

Exercise provides all kinds of benefits in addition to hot flash reduction, including the release of endorphins, a natural "upper" that enables you to put up with the signs of menopause! For optimal results, exercise thirty to forty-five minutes three to four times a week.

Try Natural/Medical and Medical Therapy

Phytoestrogens and natural progesterone in combination are discussed in chapter 17. While natural progesterone cream, lozenges, or capsules provide relief for some women, be careful about using over-the-counter natural progesterone products without investigation of their purity, dosage, manufacturing techniques, bioavailability, and risk factors.

Traditional estrogen/progestin or progesterone combinations usually work within two to six weeks and are highly effective in correcting the heat regulation disorder that causes hot flashes (see chapter 17). Their effectiveness does not justify their being the first choice if risk factors are low. However, if other interventions have not been helpful, hormone replacement therapy is justified, since unmanageable hot flashes can greatly affect the quality of one's life by interrupting sleep and by triggering depression, irritability, and the loss of a sense of well-being.

Clonidine and Megace are available by prescription. Clonidine is normally used in higher doses as an antihypertensive and in lower doses for migraine. In very low doses there has been some success in its reducing hot flashes. Research on megestrol acetate (Megace) has shown that 20 milligrams taken orally twice daily reduced the frequency of hot flashes in 85 percent of the participants after two to three weeks.[5]

When All Else Fails and You're Having a Hot Flash Now!

Try deep, paced diaphragmatic breathing. If you are able to "catch" your hot flash just as it begins, you can sometimes stop it completely, shorten it, or cause it to be milder. You are breathing correctly if your abdomen increases.

Try acupressure: Press on a point between your inner ankle-bone and Achilles tendon, three finger breadths up the leg. Press for one to three minutes when a flash begins; repeat.

Sit and with the left hand press halfway along the backside of the shoulder.

Sit and with the left hand press between the eyebrows.

Pearls of wisdom for hot flashes . . .

1. Think "Power Surge."
2. Adopt the layered look.
3. One magical cure for hot flashes does not exist. It may be necessary to experiment with multiple interventions to find the best combination for you.

5

Vulva, Vagina, and Uterus Changes

Faye left for work early, leaving the house before her husband had even gotten out of the shower. This morning she didn't have the strength to face him. Last night they had had another fight about sex—one in a series of fights that were occurring all too frequently.

Faye's resolve to "grin and bear it" simply hadn't worked, emotionally or physically. Intercourse hurt. Lovemaking left her bleeding and sore. Several months ago she had decided to begin hormones to see if they would help. If anything, her discomfort had worsened. And now she had a yeast infection that wouldn't go away.

Does any of this sound familiar? If so, read on. After seeing her doctor, Faye was able to find relief for her difficulties by using some of the suggested remedies that follow and today she is enjoying her sex life again. Before we look for solutions, however, it's good to understand just exactly what is causing all the problems.

WHAT'S CAUSING ME TO BE SO UNCOMFORTABLE?

During menopause several conditions can occur that can make sexual intercourse less pleasurable for women. Estrogen and progesterone build tissue not only in the uterus but all over the body. After menopause the outer lips of the vulva lose some of their roundedness and the inner lips become much less prominent. Doctors call this vulvar atrophy. The skin is thinner and there is

75

For the curious . . .

Changes in pH can affect the bacteria that normally live in the vagina. A delicate balance occurs between bacteria, the products they produce, estrogen, and pH levels. There are normally five to fifteen different species of bacteria living within the vagina. Around 30 percent of women with a healthy vaginal ecosystem harbor *Candida albicans,* the source of most yeast infections. When there is plenty of estrogen, and vaginal walls are thick and lush, lactobacilli are the major residents. Without it, glycogen diminishes, the pH rises, and new contaminating bacteria move in from the surrounding area such as the bowel. Itching and burning result from a chronic discharge caused by the pH elevation and the shift of bacteria in the vaginal vault.

less pubic hair. Vaginal dryness occurs because the glands providing lubrication are reduced and the mucosa becomes very thin and easily irritated. This is called urogenital atrophy.

Itching and increased susceptibility to infections occur because there are fewer cell layers, notably the surface layer which before menopause provided a tough, resilient covering. These changes affect the pH level, increasing the alkalinity and making a more favorable environment for bacteria and yeast to grow. Women who have never had problems with vaginal infections suddenly find themselves plagued with them. Accompanying these changes are problems with urgency and frequency of urination, which will be discussed in chapter 6.

With aging, the vagina becomes smaller and loses elasticity. The uterus loses mass as well. These factors, along with increased dryness, thinning walls, and small, unseen fissures, can cause painful intercourse. However, regular intercourse tends to keep the glands functional and the vaginal wall stretched, reminding us that hormones are not the only things affecting our reproductive system.

Women in midlife become more susceptible to protrusions against the vaginal wall—by the bladder (a cystocele), the rectum (a rectocele), or the intestine (an enterocele). These condi tions are dependent on the effects of previous pregnancies, disease, surgery in the pelvic area, chronic coughing due to asthma or smoking, and the degree of thinning of the vaginal wall. While all these changes may sound awful, chances are most women with mild or modest changes won't notice any difference because the majority of these signs of menopause are easily corrected or compensated for.

HEALING AN IRRITATED VAGINA

Looking at the surface may not identify many of the changes in the vagina because the source of the pain may not be readily visible. But whether the problem is visible or not, there is hope. Here are twelve natural ways to regain your vaginal health.

For the curious . . . The normal vaginal pH level is acidic, 3.8–4.2; a pH level greater than 4.5 indicates an imbalance in the vaginal ecosystem.

1. Take natural vitamin E. Vitamin E can be helpful taken orally but applying it as a cream, oil, or suppository directly to the area is often more effective. If you are using an oil-based vitamin E capsule as the source of your oil, don't simply place an unbroken capsule in the vagina. It must be broken open. Make sure the product you are using is pure and concentrated.

2. Increase intake of soy products, a rich source of isoflavones and phytosterols. Both are known to provide a mild estrogenic effect that can stimulate repair of the vaginal walls.[1]

Bacterial infections are reduced when yogurt enriched with lactobacillus acidophilus is eaten daily.[2]

3. Avoid drying substances such as antihistamines, alcohol, caffeine, and diuretics.

4. Include essential fatty acids in your diet. Make sure you get both omega-6 and omega-3 essential fatty acids (EFA). The richest source is salmon, but swordfish, mackerel, and tuna are also good, as is noninstant oatmeal eaten three to five times per week.

77

Borage oil, evening primrose oil, and flaxseed oil are wonderful sources of EFAs. For those who prefer a capsule form, we recommend either Omega EFA or EPA-DHA complex (Metagenics). More will be said about EFAs in chapter 13.

5. Drink plenty of water.

6. Wear natural fiber clothing and underwear.

7. Have regular intercourse. This increases vaginal blood flow, which facilitates repair and good health. Use a water-soluble lubricant every time you make love. KY Jelly, Astroglide, and AquaLub may help during intercourse, and longer-term moisturizers, such as Replens and GyneMoistrin, may increase daily comfort. Baby oil is not a good lubricant and may increase yeast infections.

8. Apply aluminum acetate. Acute irritation may be helped by sitz baths followed by a soothing application of aluminum acetate (Domeboro Solution).

9. Be careful of dyes, perfumes, soaps, and fabric softeners. Your more sensitive vaginal area may react to soaps, laundry detergents, vaginal contraception products, bath oils, perfumed or dyed toilet paper, and hot tub or swimming pool chemicals that did not cause allergic reactions in the past.

10. Do Kegel exercises to help maintain good vaginal and rectal muscle tone. Kegel exercises strengthen the large pubococcygeus muscle surrounding the vaginal and rectal openings. They are easily and inconspicuously done and consist of rhythmic contractions of the muscle. When contracted, the pubococcygeus muscle enables you to stop the flow of urine. Try practicing Kegels at every red light or at the beginning of every board meeting. More detail on Kegels can be found in chapter 6.

11. Try cimicifuga racemosa. Cimicifuga is an herbal extract from black cohosh. When taken orally in capsule form, it is effective in building up the vaginal mucosa.[3]

12. Try traditional Chinese herbal formulas containing roots of rehmannia and dong quai. These herbs have long been known to promote vaginal moisture.

I Think I Need Something More

If those suggestions don't correct your pain, itching, and discomfort, the following medical interventions may be helpful.

Use estrogen cream. Even among women who are taking hormone replacement orally, there is sometimes the need for additional relief of vaginal dryness and irritation. Most doctors have their preferred way of using estrogen creams, but almost all begin with a "loading" dose, tapering off to a once-a-week maintenance dose.

A typical regime might consist of 1–2 grams of estrogen cream daily for one to two weeks and then a maintenance dose once or twice a week. Small amounts of estrogen will be absorbed into the body for the first two or three weeks. As the more frequent use builds up the vaginal tissue, the amount assimilated will be negligible.

If commercial estrogen gels or creams cause further irritation, you may be allergic to the petroleum base. A pharmacist who has compounding capability can place estrogen (and phytosterols) in a water-soluble base that won't irritate. Local pharmacists and a few national pharmacies regularly make up allergy-free cream or gel bases of estradiol, estriol, or estrone, or any combination.

They can also compound natural estrogen creams (phytoestrogens), such as estriol cream (0.5 milligrams). Use 1.5 teaspoons once daily for one week, then three times a week. There is some evidence estriol may work directly on the vaginal walls. (Estriol is the weakest form of estrogen; see chapter 17.)

Think about it . . . Have you ever thought about the words we use for the vaginal area? What slang words are you aware of? None are too pretty, are they? The Chinese refer to the clitoris and vagina as "the pearl in the jade temple." What messages have you received about your vulvar area? Is it a place of beauty? Of disgust? If you don't love your vulva as much as any other part of your body, reflect for a moment on the idea of the jade temple.

79

Testosterone cream (2.5 percent) can also be compounded by a pharmacist. Apply to the labia twice daily for two weeks, then once a week for maintenance. Testosterone cream may also help with low sexual desire.

ANYTHING ELSE I CAN TRY?

Some physicians have begun to prescribe tamoxifen cream. Ten milligrams is used twice daily for four weeks for vaginal dryness.

Ciba pharmaceuticals has a relatively new estrogen patch, Vivelle, that is reputed to be particularly helpful with vaginal problems.

The first estradiol vaginal ring has now been approved. Called Estring, it is inserted into the upper portion of the vagina where it releases a consistent low dose of estrogen for three months. Upjohn and Pharmacia maintain that very little estradiol gets into the general circulation and mainly acts locally. Studies reveal it rarely causes bleeding or stimulates the endometrial lining. The ring is reported to be easy to use and is as effective as vaginal creams.

Pearls of wisdom for the jade temple . . .

1. Poor vaginal health leads to discomfort and infection. If this is a problem for you, use topical creams regularly in maintenance doses (or the new ring) to prevent problems.
2. Always use a lubricant when you have sex.

6

Bladder and Urethral Changes

"Ahh, let's see," Linda mused as she slipped a light blue cotton dress over her shoulders, straightening it out and moving back for a full view—at least as much as possible in the tiny dressing room. She went through her mental checklist, "modest neckline, long enough sleeves, length okay."

Linda's criteria were based on both real and imagined concerns. She never got around to exercising those tired triceps and for some unknown reason, she had always hated her knees. All in all, the dress seemed perfect. However, Linda hesitated and in the end decided not to purchase it. The pale blue color was lovely, but Linda was afraid that if she continued to leak urine, it would surely show. She had stopped going to her exercise class for the same reason.

Perhaps you've shared Linda's struggle with urine leakage. After spending a lifetime forgetting to go to the bathroom, midlife finds many women dealing with annoyingly increased urinary frequency. Suddenly they are getting up in the middle of the night (nocturia), or panicking that this time they will never make it to the third floor restroom, only to wait in a line of twenty-five.

Hazel, another menopausal woman, got so self-conscious about her leakage that she was convinced anyone who got close to her would smell urine. She gave up walking with her friends because she interrupted their pace with her bathroom stops.

Linda and Hazel didn't have to make such concessions. Problems with stress incontinence, such as leaking urine when one laughs, coughs, or exercises, can be annoying, but they are relatively easy to remedy. It is estimated that six million women between the ages of thirty-five and sixty-five have stress incontinence, and only one out of twelve consults a physician. For many women, it is simply a bothersome accompaniment to menopause.

Changes in the vulvar area are due to decreased levels of estrogen. But there is some evidence that a previous hysterectomy or current obesity increase the odds of developing incontinence. The breakdown is a mechanical one, which secondarily increases the odds of infection. A bladder infection always needs proper evaluation and medical treatment. Our focus is keeping the area healthy so infections will be minimal and urinary leakage will not limit any woman from living the lifestyle she desires.

WHY CAN'T I PASS A BATHROOM WITHOUT STOPPING?

Do bathrooms hold a fascination for you that they haven't had since you were potty trained? The reason is relatively simple. Both the lower urinary and genital tracts share a common origin and are equally subject to the effects of estrogen. Since estrogen acts directly on the urethra—affecting its physical dimensions, vascular supply, and enervation—when the estrogen supply decreases, urinary changes are inevitable.[1] Just as with the tissue in the vagina and the surrounding area, during menopause, urinary tract tissue becomes thinner and less elastic. When there was plenty of estrogen-sensitive epithelium, it contributed to closing off the urethra through its well-nourished nerves and surrounding tissue.

For the curious . . . Most normal adult women urinate six to eight times per day and may get up to go to the bathroom from zero to one time at night.

Lack of estrogen causes the area between the vagina and the urethra to shrink. As the vagina shortens and narrows, the urethral opening tilts closer to the vaginal opening making activities such as coitus, douching, inserting a vaginal preparation, or even sitting on a narrow bicycle seat the source of an inflamed urethra (urethritis) and/or inflamed bladder (cystitis).

For the curious . . .
There are five types of incontinence. Which describes yours?
1. Urge Incontinence
   - Strong urge to urinate
   - Urination occurs more frequently
   - Nighttime trips to the bathroom
   - May have little urine
2. Stress Incontinence
   - Loss of small amount of urine when coughing, laughing, sneezing, straining
   - Usually do not have to get up at night
3. Functional Incontinence
   - Early morning incontinence
   - Accidents on the way to the bathroom
4. Overflow Incontinence
   - Swollen bladder
   - Tenderness above pubic region
   - Reduced urine flow
5. Iatrogenic Incontinence
   - Sudden changes in urinary pattern after surgery or new medication

To the naked eye, the whole area may appear normal despite these changes. Other types of incontinence, not especially related to menopause, are caused by degeneration of nerve pathways due to aging, diabetes, multiple sclerosis, and so forth.

WHAT TO DO

1. Exercise the pelvic floor with Kegel exercises. If done correctly, they effectively control urine leakage by maintaining good muscle tone. See "For the curious . . ." on the next page.

For the curious . . .

How to do pelvic floor exercises (Kegels)

1. Tighten the muscles of the pelvic floor; hold for 3–4 seconds; relax (sustained contraction).
2. Follow with three quick contractions in succession; relax (intermittent contraction).
3. Repeat steps 1 and 2 ten times, while sitting and standing.
4. Do not hold your breath.
5. Use only pelvic muscles; avoid tightening thighs or buttocks.
6. Feel abdominal muscles; avoid bearing down and pushing instead of tightening.
7. Repeat three times per day.

To test if you are doing Kegels correctly, try to halt urination before you are empty. *Only* do this as a test, not to train yourself. To understand what you are *not* to do, hold your breath and push down with your abdomen, as if you were having a bowel movement.

2. Lubricants during sex reduce the chance of tearing and trauma to delicate tissue. Sex itself keeps the area in good condition. Get in the habit of always applying a lubricant before having sex.

3. It may help to take vitamin E orally or rub it directly on the vulva.

4. Watch your weight. Studies show that being 25 percent overweight increases problems of urinary incontinence because of increased pressure from above on the pelvic structures.

5. Control over the urge to urinate can be taught and the bladder can be trained to empty at set times. It involves controlling fluid intake while gradually increasing the time between urination until there are three hours between voiding. A physician can give you specific details and determine if such training would be beneficial for you.

6. Estrogen cream used the same way as recommended for vaginal dryness improves urinary control (see chapter 5).[2] Treatment with low-potency estrogen, such as estriol, has been shown to be effective and is a common choice in Europe. It is considered to be a "weak" estrogen and possibly anticarcinogenic. Estradiol is the most biologically active form of estrogen and when given in low doses helps thicken urogenital tissue without affecting other estrogen-sensitive areas.

7. Estring, developed for vaginal dryness, fits directly in the vagina and is also effective for urogenital symptoms and atrophy (see chapter 5).

8. Oral or transdermal estrogen may be needed in addition to vaginal application. If the concern is for urogenital problems only, even very low doses delivered through a skin patch have been helpful.[3] While such a low dose does not reduce the risk of cardiovascular disease and osteoporosis, it does help with urogenital problems without the risk of vaginal bleeding or other estrogenic effects elsewhere in the body.

9. Keep up on all the current information about incontinence on the Internet.

HOW DO I KNOW IF I NEED SURGERY?

Functional urethral changes due to menopause rarely require surgery. However, many women begin urine leakage as a result of damage from childbearing and resultant changes in their pelvic/vaginal anatomy, or due to neurological changes from nerve injury in childbirth or the result of disease such as diabetes that manifests for the first time at menopause. Or you may have a cystocele, a condition where the weakened bladder floor bulges downward pushing against the upper vaginal wall.

Some urinary problems can be caused by medication. Careful evaluation is necessary to determine the source of your problem. Should it be anatomical in origin, you may, indeed, need surgery. But never undergo surgery before having a comprehensive evaluation that spells out the risks, confirms the diagnosis, and lets you know how your quality of life will be affected. If you aren't ready to face surgery, there are several devices designed to support the bladder neck:

- The bladder neck support prosthesis is worn during the day with 83 percent efficacy. It is removed at night. It costs less than four hundred dollars.
- Incontinence rings can be fitted to support the bladder neck. They are removable and cost thirty to forty dollars.
- New treatments using collagen injections offer some promise. The long-term risks and benefits are as yet unknown.
- An all-male research team must have invented two other new treatments. One involves placing tape over the urethral opening, removing as needed. The other is a balloon-like device that is inserted into the urethral opening and inflated. It must be deflated to urinate.

Pearls of wisdom about avoiding bladder infections . . .

1. Drink lots of fluids.
2. Drink cranberry juice daily.
3. Take vitamin C.
4. Avoid sugar and refined carbohydrates.

2

Skin and Mucous Membranes

As if there weren't enough to deal with at midlife, women suddenly find their skin more troublesome than it's been since age fifteen. While the teen years were plagued with excess oil, most midlife women struggle to keep their skin from looking as if they have done nothing more with their life than sunbathe. And ironically, for a few, acne again becomes a problem.

The primary skin change related to declining estrogen is the reduction of collagen. Collagen is the main supportive protein of not only skin but bone, cartilage, and connective tissue. As skin and mucous membranes lose their resilience due to reduction in collagen thickness, a transformation in appearance occurs. This is due to changes in collagen and blood vessels. Most women are well aware of the metamorphosis normally attributed to aging, which includes wrinkling, drying, thinning, mutations in pigment, and reduced elasticity.

As we age, our thinning blood vessel walls lead to increased bruising. It is not uncommon to inadvertently redecorate your aging mother with incriminating fingerprint-like bruises just by helping her in or out of a car or chair. To make matters worse, healing time is doubled because of the slowed epidermis turnover rate.

Changes unrelated to decreasing estrogen and related more to the way you have lived accentuate the development of a variety of "age or brown spots" (actinic keratosis). Sunscreen can help in preventing them, and they can be removed by freezing (cryosurgery), laser treatments, or similar ablative methods. Many dermatologists advise that it is simply best to live with our spots. We can help them fade by staying out of the sun.

For the curious . . . During the first five years after the menopause, 30 percent of the skin collagen is lost. Collagen is what keeps skin toned and wrinkle free.

The skin reveals more lines and less tone as we age because the underlying support has been reduced. Loss of collagen and elasticity is readily evident in our "expression" lines. Decreased thickness also means fewer oil glands in the skin—less oil, more dryness. Even the mouth can become dry. Due to the changing hormonal levels, hair thins and dries on the head, while defiantly increasing on the face.

Fewer oil glands and dry skin make us feel "itchy." Some menopausal women are even plagued by a feeling of something crawling on their skin. Others complain their skin becomes hypersensitive, necessitating adjustments in the way they are comfortable being touched.

NATURE'S DIRTY LITTLE BEAUTY TRICK

If your dermatologist is also your best friend, he or she has let you know that a simple trip outside must be a major preventative operation. Hats, sunblock, long sleeves, and gloves must be religiously worn, and the cover-up complete and consistent. Are all dermatologists alarmists, with controlling personalities, or do they know something we don't? In truth, we know it too. We just don't pay attention.

We seek, instead, great-looking tans. There are few things as deceptive. How something so damaging can look so healthy is one of the monumental mysteries of life. Exposure to the sun can cause problems of fine superficial lines on the skin's surface, blotchiness, and even cancerous growths. In fact sun damage is the real culprit in skin aging even more than heredity or loss of estrogen. While protecting ourselves from the sun continues to be important as we age, it is the cumulative lifetime damage of sun rays, weather, and pollutants that finally catches up with us. At fifty it is almost too late to follow our dermatologist's advice. Not so for our daughters, although getting them to listen when we didn't is a challenge.

As tedious as it seems, you must make applying sunblock as routine as brushing your teeth. Choose products that have an SPF number of 15 or more and protect from both UVA and UVB rays. Today many moisturizers and makeups have sun protection included. A titanium dioxide sunblock is less likely to sting eyes. Don't limit your application to your face. Remember your arms and backs of your hands. If the tan look is still the rage in your area, use the new improved self-tanners. Dermatologists tell us they work on the surface and are safe as long as you remember they are not sunblocks. Tanning salons are not recommended. They are no safer than sitting in the sun.

GOLF BALLS, WRINKLES, AND SMOKE

The most leathery, wrinkled skin seen at our clinic is on women who smoke and spend hours in the sun golfing. The combination is unrelenting in its damage. Years of sun exposure combined with smoke by-products thicken and harden the skin, leaving it deeply furrowed. Cigarette smoking alone changes skin. It reduces circulation by decreasing the capillary blood flow, and therefore reduces cell nutrition. Externally, it leaves a toxic film on the face. Among Caucasian women, this combination results in two to three times the number of facial wrinkles as on a woman who doesn't smoke.

Other habits affect skin health as well, such as consuming too much caffeine or alcohol, which robs the body of water and interferes with absorption of nutrients. Not supplying the necessary nutrition because of poor diet and not drinking enough water (eight 6–8-ounce glasses per day) are big factors in aging skin.

The point is, because of the loss of estrogen and consequent reduction in collagen, women at midlife can no longer get away with the kinds of things they assumed they were getting away with in their youth. Dry indoor environments, harsh soaps, poor diets, and most of all sunlight combine to escalate the skin's aging capacity. More important, they increase its susceptibility to skin cancer.

AVOIDING THOSE CRACKS AND CREVICES

There are several things you can do to lessen the effects of midlife changes on your skin.

1. Exercise. Improved circulation nourishes skin and helps it stay healthy from the inside.

2. Add essential oils to your diet (see chapter 13).

3. Reduce stress. Stress causes blood to be sent to vital organs like the brain and heart and to bypass the skin. The result is a pale, ashen look and under-eye circles. Stress also tells the adrenal glands to release hormones that increase sebaceous gland secretions and cause skin to break out.

4. Try new products. Despite manufacturers' claims, until the last few years, other than sunblock, there were no products on the market that truly reduced wrinkles. Today there are several that actually work. Weak versions can be purchased over the counter, but our recommendation is to consult a dermatologist.

Alpha-hydroxy acid products promise to reduce lines and age spots. This acid occurs naturally in fruits and is an exfoliator, sweeping away dead surface cells to reveal smoother, softer skin underneath. A 5 percent strength is usually enough and it can be used in conjunction with retin-A. Do not waste your money purchasing products with AHA that are rinse-off versions, since they must have continued contact with the skin to be effective. Their effect lasts only as long as they are used.

Retin-A, topical retinoids (vitamin A derivatives), can improve skin texture and eradicate fine lines when applied regularly over a period of months. It works by decreasing the cohesiveness of epidermal cells, which allows them to slough off more easily so that a smoother skin texture results.

5. Chemical peels remove the epidermis but penetrate deeper to improve fine lines, skin texture, and skin color. This should only be done by a qualified dermatologist. The new Fluor-Hydroxy Pulse (pulse peel) destroys precancerous cells without hurting normal ones, while also helping cosmetically.

6. Try vitamin C. Over-the-counter products, such as Cellex-C, are used topically to counteract environmental damage. Vitamin C stimulates collagen synthesis and may act as a natural sunscreen. It is the only vitamin with proven effects on the skin—500-C methoxyflavone (Metagenics) has proven effective in preventing bruising.

7. Choose soap wisely. All soap is irritating. Unscented Dove is widely available and the least irritating to a large number of people, including those who suffer from acne. If it doesn't work for you, try Aveenobar (made of oatmeal), Purpose, Basis, or Oil of Olay Cleansing Bar.

8. Avoid very hot water. Take one shower a day, for less than five minutes, with water on the cool side. People with very sensitive skin may find even this is too much.

9. Apply lotions. Lotions make us feel and smell good but to be most effective they should be applied immediately after a bath to trap the moisture that is on the skin. Nutraderm, Purpose, Moistural, or DML lotions can be purchased over the counter and are effective. If needed, they can be applied several times during the day. If your skin is extremely dry, you can try Aveeno Moisturizing Cream or DML Forte. Sensitive skin may react to lotions containing lanolin, aloe vera, and fragrance.

10. Be careful with fabric softeners. While most laundry detergents can be used as long as rinse cycles are adequate, many women react, especially in the vulvar-vaginal area, to fabric softeners, especially those used in the dryer. "Static cling" products are bothersome for some women.

11. Consider hormone replacement (see chapter 17). While some women have found natural progesterone creams and/or triestrogen products helpful, the most effective treatment for maintaining collagen in the skin and bones is traditional hormone replacement. Studies have demonstrated improvement in skin thickness, fine wrinkling, and tone in women who take hormones. There is a correlation between the time since menopause and the amount of collagen lost. This points to an advantage in beginning estrogen early to maintain collagen levels.

12. Herbs and foods that contain phytoestrogens and antioxidants may protect connective tissue by improving the detoxification of waste products and preventing free radical damage to the skin.

An important pearl of wisdom for the nicest skin . . .

Staying out of the sun is the most significant thing you can do for skin health.

8

Fatigue and Sleeplessness

Janet unlocked the door to her condo, threw the keys on the hutch, tossed her purse in the closet, and went straight upstairs. She didn't bother to undress, check her messages, or read the mail. Within minutes she was asleep and she didn't stir until her friend Olivia called to remind her they were due at a meeting in half an hour.

Janet was worried. She had always been a dynamo, pushing and driving those around her to produce more. She had always led the pack. No one worked harder, did more, or seemed more passionate about life than Janet. Dragging around was not her style. In fact she had felt somewhat contemptuous of those who had to slow down and take a breath between projects. Since James died, the void had been filled with even greater busyness. It just wasn't normal for her to be so tired.

She was sure something was physically wrong. She assumed that her doctor would give her a pill and everything would be fine. But other than an FSH score that indicated she was flirting with menopause, lab tests gave no clue as to the source of her overwhelming fatigue. But Janet was lucky. Her doctor took enough time to get a sense of her lifestyle, being well aware of some important midlife issues Janet had yet to face.

HELP, I'M FALLING ASLEEP AT THE WHEEL

Women like Janet, whose lives have been perpetual motion, often make their way to a physician's office when they discover they can no longer continue as they always have. In fact this is so common that it is the explanation given for why so many more women who use hormones tend to be white, middle class, and well-educated. Such women have found their way to the doctor's office because they have insurance and are unwilling to put up with factors that limit their ability to function as usual.

Fatigue is one of the top five reasons people see doctors, and a major reason midlife women make an appointment. While it may be a symptom of a serious illness, it is more often a reflection of an exhausting lifestyle. There are few people today who are not being asked to work harder and play less. Downsizing, overtime, shrinking vacations, and no opportunity to pace oneself due to the onslaught of e-mail, faxes, pagers, and cell phones make today's pace faster than at any other time in history. The result is there is no down time, no time to think about a response when someone is waiting for an immediate reply.

Less restorative sleep, overstimulation, minimal-to-no exercise, and ever increasing responsibility associated with work, home, kids, and aging parents require more energy than our bodies can produce. Waking up tired can be a sign of chronic illness as well as a psychological and/or spiritual struggle.

**Think about it . . .
As a woman, whether you work in or out of the home, the tendency is to put the needs of others first. Perhaps for the first time in your life, you feel unable to continue your caretaking pattern. Ask yourself two questions:
1. Why should I?
2. What do I need to keep mentally and physically healthy?**

There are many causes for exhaustion. Grieving over losses—elderly parents losing their minds, divorce, or missed opportunities—makes us feel tired. Conflicts over trying to be everything to everybody plague women throughout their lives and sometimes are challenged for the first time at midlife. Depression, though not more common in midlife women, can also explain fatigue. Until the underlying issues are dealt with, tremendous energy is expended, trying to cope and keep going.

Chinese medicine looks at fatigue as being an imbalance of qi (pronounced chee), loosely translated as life energy or vitality. When exhausted, the body is believed to have expended its energy or potential. Western medicine speaks of burned-out adrenals and faulty endocrine or hormonal systems. In any case, focusing on one's overall health is generally the most important thing that can be done for fatigue.

WHEN THE MACHINE BREAKS DOWN

Janet slept when she was exhausted. Others speak of "hitting the wall" or going through the motions as if on autopilot. Still others become weepy and overwhelmed. Biologically, exhaustion means that the body has depleted its energy sources, causing an accumulation of waste products, which inhibit production of more energy. The problem is twofold: chemical imbalance from overexertion followed by a breakdown in regulation between the communication systems that coordinate nervous and endocrine systems. If you are preoccupied with your fatigue, take that as an indication that it is out of control.

DO I HAVE CHRONIC FATIGUE?

Fatigue that keeps us from completing tasks is common, but chronic fatigue is not. Rest does not relieve chronic fatigue, and the person who has it can only manage a very low level of activity. Short-term memory and the ability to concentrate are impaired. Chronic fatigue is accompanied by a sore throat, painful lymph nodes, muscle pain, joint pain, headache, and sleep disturbance lasting more than six months.

Building up the immune system is an important part of recovery. Because it is such a prolonged and debilitating disease, psychological support is helpful. A study from Britain demonstrated the effect of cognitive therapy on chronic fatigue. People who underwent four months of counseling to help them understand the illness, have patience with a slow recovery, and overcome mental blocks were more likely to return to normal functioning after twelve months than those who had no therapy (73 percent versus 27 percent). Counseling was helpful, not a cure, but its effect was substantial. The emphasis on understanding the disease and what can be done about it proved most effective.

If you think you may be suffering from chronic fatigue or something close to it, accept that your recovery is likely to be slow. Examine your lifestyle. Do you overextend yourself physically or emotionally? With your doctor's assistance and approval, begin an elimination diet (a diet low in allergens) to uncover foods to which you have a reaction. Stay on the diet for at least three weeks before reintroducing banned foods, one at a time.

Recent studies show that improving gastrointestinal health through diet, detox, and programmed nutrition improves chronic health problems.[1] Select highly digestible sources of protein and use digestive enzymes. Eat balanced meals that include all food groups. Limit your aerobic activity; walking is a good choice. Build strength by light weight lifting. Take a high-potency nutritional supplement (see appendix B), and for additional therapy add 200–300 milligrams of magnesium three times a day, 500–1,000 milligrams of vitamin C three times a day, 50–150 milligrams of coenzyme Q10, and 1 tablespoon of an essential fatty acid such as flaxseed oil or one GLA Forte capsule daily (Metagenics). Use herbs such as milk thistle *(Silybum marianum)*, garlic, Siberian ginseng, echinacea, and/or some of the traditional Chinese combinations recommended for liver and adrenal support (see chapter 20).

WHAT ELSE KEEPS ME TIRED?

Take a look in your medicine cabinet. Got allergies? Got antihistamines? Chances are you may be using the new antihistamines guaranteed not to make you sleepy during the day—which, like the television bunny, "keep on working" through the night, keeping you up. Make sure the effect has worn off by evening or use an old-fashioned version that leaves you bleary-eyed and asleep by the evening news. Other medications that cause fatigue are analgesics, salicylates, antidepressants, antihypertensives, beta-blockers, muscle relaxants, and sedatives.

If your bleeding pattern has been heavy, do not rule out the possibility that anemia is the cause of your fatigue. Women with severe bleeding develop iron deficiency anemia.

Food allergies are major but overlooked culprits that steal your energy. Dairy products and sugar are particularly suspect. Don't overlook the possibility of your unique reaction to certain foods.

Adrenal overdrive (see chapter 20) can also leave you worn out, as well as affecting your ovarian and thyroid function. Feeling tired is a classic symptom of low thyroid function. Overgrowth of yeast and/or a parasitic infection in the intestinal tract may also be the source. And don't forget the possibility of toxins in your system (see chapter 20). This is a lesson I learned the hard way, as I explained in the introduction.

EATING FOR ENERGY

Just as your car can't run without fuel and runs poorly with bad fuel, your body can't function with inadequate nutrients or erratic delivery. A consistent, high quality fuel supply in the form of frequent, nutritious small meals and snacks will help keep you going. This pattern is the opposite of what you do when dieting. Your energy level is affected by what you eat because it is your food that supplies the fuel for the brain to keep you vital and alert (see chapter 13 for more information).

INCREASING YOUR ENERGY LEVEL

1. Choose exercise over food. Exercise burns calories and boosts energy. It provides fitness and endurance and increases the efficiency of the lungs, thereby increasing blood oxygen levels. It contributes to the body's ability to remove waste products, keeps the nervous system running, speeds up the metabolism, and is a mood enhancer because of increased endorphin production.

2. Take supplements. A daily multivitamin is often necessary because good diets are sometimes spoiled by food handling and pesticide exposure. Remember, both a deficiency of vitamins and an excess of vitamins can cause fatigue, so avoid megadoses as well as not getting enough essential vitamins. Excess fat soluble vitamins, such as A, D, E, and K, are not flushed out of the body, so don't overdo them.

If heavy bleeding is a problem, consider a supplement with iron and folic acid. If you've stopped having periods, you probably do not need additional iron, which has been shown to have a negative effect on the heart. Iron can also be obtained in the diet by eating raisins, dark leafy greens, beans, or herbs, such as yellow dock, dandelion, nettles, burdock, or mullein leaves (see chapter 13 for more nutritional information).

B vitamins, pantothenic acid (B5), vitamin C, magnesium, potassium, and tyrosine can help stressed-out adrenals. Siberian ginseng helps with fatigue, but be aware that too much can cause bleeding. Licorice root extract stimulates the adrenal and causes the adrenal hormone cortisol to be effective longer. It combats stress caused by overwork and poor nutrition. However, it should be used only temporarily and not at all if you are hypertensive or have other cardiovascular disease. If using licorice root alone, be certain it contains a standardized amount of glycyrrhizen. Do not exceed 400 milligrams of glycyrrhizen per day.

3. Stabilize your blood sugar. Make carbohydrate food choices from low-glycemic foods like vegetables and fruits that enter your system slowly, rather than large doses of dense carbohydrates such as donuts, cookies, pasta, and breads. Eat small meals more frequently and include a balance of carbohydrates, proteins, and a little fat. Protein foods provide energy by prompting the body to produce more glucagon. Eating too much protein is not the way to gain more energy—eating in balance is (see chapter 13).

4. Keep a record of your fatigue pattern. Not only will you be better able to handle fatigue related to food, but you may discover "psychological lows" that are related to tasks or people you must deal with.

5. Don't underestimate the importance of drinking enough water. Dehydration is exhausting. Drink twice as much water as your thirst dictates.

6. Stop smoking. Nicotine may either stimulate the brain so it uses excessive energy or depress brain function by causing an increased need for oxygen in the bloodstream. A person who has recently quit smoking gets more tired because of the loss of the

short-term stimulating effect. Nicotine works in the same way as alcohol, which at first stimulates and then acts as a depressant.

I KNOW WHY I'M TIRED—I DON'T SLEEP!

Mary never had any trouble going to sleep. But, like clock-work, she was wide awake at 2:30 A.M. Tracy tossed and turned and when she did drift off would awaken with the slightest noise. Doreen dreaded each night as wave upon wave of hot flashes and night sweats left her close to tears, miserable, and frustrated. Myrna slept but not "like a rock" as she had in the past. During the day she had trouble concentrating and had been plagued by a series of accidents.

There are a lot of patterns of sleeplessness during the peri-menopause and menopause but they have one thing in common—they make life miserable. We know from wartime experiences and scientific studies, not to mention horror movies, that sleep deprivation can undermine the strongest resolve and make one feel as if counting flowers on the wall of a very small room in a "special" place is the next inevitable step.

The truth is that even a small disruption in the length of sleep time or the depth of sleep can profoundly affect our moods and efficiency. Yet all Americans sleep less than they did in the past, according to the Sleep Disorders Center at Emory University. At thirty-five, our parents snoozed eight to nine hours a night. Now we are lucky to get seven or eight hours, with one person in four getting even less. Perhaps this is the explanation for why we are fatter than ever, since animal studies reveal that animals who get less sleep eat more! Not sleeping can cause you to be nervous and forgetful and make it difficult for you to take care of your respon-sibilities or, like Myrna, be accident prone. Physically it can cause heart and digestive problems.

HOW MANY SHEEP DO I HAVE TO COUNT BEFORE I KNOW I HAVE A PROBLEM?

Anyone who regularly is unable to fall asleep in thirty minutes or who wakes up after a few hours and can't go back to sleep is said to have insomnia. Normal sleep occurs in cycles, usually five per night, lasting about ninety minutes each. In four of these cycles our metabolism and brain wave rate slow down. During this time the body physically grows, tissue is repaired, and immune functions occur.

One of the five cycles is REM (rapid eye movement) in which body activity picks up and we dream. It is having this cycle disrupted that causes many of the difficulties we have when awake. In other words, it is not simply the amount of time we sleep, but the quality of sleep that is important. When we are deprived of REM sleep we become anxious, irritable, and have difficulty concentrating. Our immune system suffers when REM is in short supply. Sleep aids given to midlife women generally do not help because even if they induce sleep, they do not trigger this restorative cycle.

Many diseases and medications affect sleep. For example, poor thyroid function can cause fitful sleep and daytime fatigue if it is not producing enough hormone (hypothyroidism). On the other hand, if the thyroid is churning out too much hormone, it causes wakefulness due to anxiety and a racing heart (hyperthyroidism). Overstimulation of the central nervous system due to hypothalamic disturbances can result in very patterned awakenings.

KNOCK ME OUT, PLEASE

What can you do to change your present sleep maladies? Here are some worthwhile suggestions.

1. Try aromatherapy. Scientific data has now proven the effectiveness of lavender oil in a bath, on a lamp, dabbed on the pillow, or dried by the bedside as a sleep aid.

2. Control hot flashes. Sleeplessness is often second only to hot flashes as the symptom sending women for medical help (see chapter 4 for how to deal with hot flashes).

3. Watch for depression. Sleeping fitfully, particularly with early-morning awakenings, may be related to depression. Specifically, depression alters sleep patterns causing more awakenings from which you are unable to go back to sleep and less deep sleep (see chapter 9 on depression).

4. Consider your diet and eat a snack before bedtime. Caffeine and alcohol both stimulate, but alcohol also depresses. Alcohol may cause a person to fall asleep but wake up during the night. Warm milk and tuna contain tryptophan, an amino acid that acts as a sedative since it is a precursor to serotonin. Snack on foods rich in tryptophan such as milk, yogurt, turkey, almonds, bananas, tuna, or peanut butter before bedtime. They will not only relax you but help you maintain your blood sugar throughout the night.

5. Get enough exercise. Little children rarely have trouble sleeping. Try following their pattern of staying active. Exercise early in the day to avoid energizing yourself at night when you want to be slowing down.

6. Try supplements such as vitamins B3, B6, and B12. Calcium and magnesium, in a 2 to 1 ratio, calm the nervous system. Niacinamide (1 gram at bedtime) will help stimulate serotonin and promote sleep.

7. Try herbs as teas and tinctures. Saint-John's-wort, valerian, hops, passion flower, and chamomile are effective for some people at bedtime and do not affect the central nervous system as do prescription drugs.

8. Do something that requires brain power. Ever wonder why, after a long day of just thinking, you can be so tired? Mental activity uses considerable calories and increases the amount of good REM sleep.

9. Consider whether medication is the problem. Prescription and over-the-counter drugs often cause sleeplessness, so read package inserts to see if you are experiencing a drug side effect.

10. Reduce physical pain. Aches and pains can interrupt sleep by making you uncomfortable and restless and by increasing cortisol levels—our fight-or-flight response. An aspirin before bed may serve to aid sleep and heart health at the same time, or better yet, try a natural muscle relaxant such as Myoplex PM or, for acute pain, Inflavonoid (both from Metagenics).

11. Consider checking your adrenal function. Persons with fibromyalgia and arthritis usually have stimulated the adrenal gland for so long that it is fatigued (see chapter 20).

12. Make sure your bladder is empty. Watch your fluid consumption before bedtime.

13. Take a warm bath. Warm baths, containing aromatic herbs and oils that aid sleep, can be very helpful. Or try a bath with Epsom salts to ease muscle aches and pain. If you are having trouble with hot flashes at night, do not take your bath just before bed. The heat from the bath will trigger hot flashes and interfere with your sleep.

14. Try melatonin—temporarily. You may find a temporary, small dose, 1–3 milligrams or less, of melatonin helpful to reestablish sleep patterns either for the short or long term.

15. Take hormones. Hormone replacement therapy has been proven to positively affect sleep-related respiratory disturbances that tend to increase at midlife, such as apnea, slow interrupted breathing, and low oxygen levels in the blood.[2] After six weeks of hormone use, sleep-lab testing of women, comparing patterns before and after HRT, showed an almost one-third increase in REM sleep time, a lowering of the mean heart rate while sleeping, and improvement in total sleep time and sleep efficiency. Menopausal women who acted as controls were not given HRT and did not improve and were shown to have abnormally low cerebral blood flow, which fell even lower during hot flashes.[3]

In a very short time hormones can be very helpful for a variety of sleep problems. Taking HRT at night, when food is less likely to affect its bioavailability and thus stabilize its level, insures the greatest impact on hot flashes and night sweats. Since progesterone has a known sedative quality, it is recommended it be taken at night. (Natural progesterone is sometimes taken twice a day with the larger dose at night.)

DISCOVER GOOD SLEEP HYGIENE

Scientists who study sleep lecture about the importance of "sleep hygiene." They aren't referring to the number of showers you take or how often you change the linen. They are referring to habits and patterns that affect sleep. For example, taking daytime naps may be interfering with falling asleep at night; so may using your bed as a desk from which you do your work or read, maybe even watch TV. If you have sleep problems, reserve the bed for sleeping and sex.

Clean up your act by going to bed and getting up at the same time, even on days you don't have to. Regulate your room temperature and avoid extremes, providing a dark and quiet environment. Exercise, but not right before bedtime. Instead, establish a nice bedtime ritual that is relaxing and provides "cues" to go to sleep. This is especially important if you have conditioned yourself to become anxious about whether or not you will fall asleep. If sleep is not achieved in thirty minutes, get up, read, or do something boring until you feel sleepy. Don't toss and turn.

There is so much more known about sleep now than just a few years ago. If none of the above has given you relief, most cities have physician-operated sleep centers for an in-depth look at your problem. There are now twelve categories of sleep disorders and fifty-five subheadings as of the 1990 International Classification of Sleep Disorders. Here are some of them:

- *Sleep apnea* is a breathing disorder that disrupts sleep and is known to increase in menopausal women.
- *Periodic limb movement* also becomes more prevalent with age and keeps people up by causing twitches and jerks that prevent the sleeper from entering REM restorative patterns.
- *Restless leg syndrome* is often genetic in origin and a more complex form of periodic limb movement.
- *Subjective insomnia* involves anxiety about not sleeping. Often we are actually sleeping more than we think we are, even when we are often checking the clock. If you feel good and refreshed in the morning and are not dozing during the day, you are probably getting enough sleep.
- *Sleep maintenance insomnia* means you wake up and are unable to go back to sleep. Menopausal women may awaken due to hot flashes, crawling skin sensations, or joint and muscle pain. Insomnia may also be due to cortisol output and blood sugar dips (hypoglycemia) at night.

TURN ON THE LIGHTS!

Occasionally problems with sleep are because our natural biological rhythms are out of sync. For instance, you may have gotten into the habit of going to bed later and later. Melatonin may be helpful in slowly resetting your clock, but you can also retrain your body by going to bed slightly earlier each night and gradually rolling back your bedtime. Using bright lights when you come home from work and then soft lighting an hour or two before going to bed in a very dark room sometimes helps reset your circadian or natural body rhythm. Use light and exercise to help get your body going in the morning.

Pearls of wisdom for sleeping and fatigue . . .

1. Sleep problems are a common symptom of menopause but they can have a multiple origin.
2. Fatigue is also a common menopause complaint but multiple factors may also be at work.
3. "Playing" until you are tired is a great sleep enhancer.

Memory, Mood Swings, and Depression

For many women in midlife, disruption of the emotional side of their lives—the perception of being slightly out of control accompanied by the loss of a sense of well-being—is more distressing than physical discomforts. It certainly was for Noreen. It was her failing memory that brought her into her doctor's office, not hot flashes.

On more than one occasion, Noreen had found herself forgetting where she was going. Once she had ended up in a strange neighborhood. She'd had to pull over and calm herself, then systematically recall the series of events that had placed her on the corner of Lock and North Streets. She finally did remember, but the whole experience was unnerving. The day before her appointment, she hadn't been able to recall her best friend's phone number. The day before that, she couldn't recollect any of her cards in her weekly bridge class. She was convinced that the proverbial "Home for the Bewildered" was only a step away.

Despite her fear, Noreen was not losing her mind or on her way to full-fledged dementia. She was menopausal. As her estrogen levels fell, the rate and efficiency of communication between synapses and dendrites in the brain were diminishing, and her memory suffered.

Forgetting, as annoying as it is, is not life threatening. The lower levels of estrogen that may be contributing to forgetting do not necessarily demand hormone replacement. Mental functioning, like some of the other signs of menopause, frequently evens out

105

For the curious . . .

The hippocampus contains estrogen receptors and is the part of the brain concerned with learning and memory. It is highly affected by estrogen levels. Concentrations of neurotransmitters are influenced by estrogen, particularly the neurotransmitter acetylcholine, the depletion of which is connected with memory loss.

Good memory is the result of a combination of actions within the brain. Estrogen has a specific function and adequate amounts result in better performance by enhancing short-term verbal memory and the ability to learn new material.[1] Inability to remember words and names of items or people is a sign of waning estrogen.[2] Having to work to remember familiar and common terms was worrisome to Noreen, as it would be for anyone who experienced it. Estrogen does not affect general attention or visual/spatial memory, but there is some evidence that progesterone may improve both.[3]

over time. However, if your risk factors allow it and your symptoms are annoying enough, hormone replacement will help.

According to a 1996 study from the UCLA School of Medicine, menopausal women had strikingly improved scores on mental performance and brain image activity when they started on estrogen.[4] Improvement occurred generally and reflected a 22 percent increase in activity in the cerebral cortex. This resulted in improved short-term and verbal memory. New brain scan procedures using tomography give visual proof of increased blood flow and activity.

Premarin, an estrogen replacement, contains an ingredient associated with learning and memory—equilin—and contains less 17 beta-estradiol that reportedly inhibits temporal lobe nerve cell growth.[5]

THINGS THAT WILL HELP YOU REMEMBER

Helpful as they are, however, hormones are not a "mental tonic" that will fix all that is missing from your memory. While you are waiting for your body to adjust, or need a boost in addition to your estrogen, you may want to try the following:

1. Ginkgo. This is a popular, safe herb derived from the world's oldest living tree species, the *Ginkgo biloba*. It has been used in Chinese medicine and extensively in Europe to improve blood flow to the brain and enhance energy production. Its effectiveness has been demonstrated in a number of scientific tests.

While ginkgo is available in many health food stores, make sure what you buy is standardized and contains 24 percent ginkgo flavonglycosides. A 40–80-milligram capsule can be taken up to three times a day. Most people see improvement within two to four weeks, with increasing improvement over time. There have been no problems reported with long-term use at this dose. Side effects are very rare, but mild gastrointestinal upset and headache are possible.

2. Maintain your blood sugar. Like any engine that supplies the power to the rest of the machine, the brain requires a constant supply of oxygen (20 percent of your total supply) and nutrients and glucose for fuel, so it is important to eat regularly. When glucose is in short supply, it can cause "foggy" thinking, marked fatigue, and mood changes (see chapter 13).

3. Eat a balanced diet. Because the brain is so active, it needs nearly every vitamin and mineral known. A variety of nutrients are utilized to help build neurotransmitters that are essential for the transfer of information from nerve cell to nerve cell. Memory is directly related to the speed at which nerve impulses can be transmitted. The faster the impulse, the better your memory.

For the curious . . . Estrogen enriches the hippocampus and increases choline acetyl-transferase and the efficiency of nerve synapses.

4. Rule out atherosclerotic plaque. Have your doctor check your carotid arteries to evaluate the extent the blood flows to the brain. An ultrasound machine measures the amount of blood flow and reveals the degree of blockage present.

I Just Want to Feel Like I Used To!

Patricia found the signs of menopause mildly annoying but tolerable, except for her psychological volatility. It was something new and it scared her. She was a big, friendly woman, whom everybody loved. For a brief time she had worked as a nursery school teacher but most of her life had been spent as a "professional" volunteer, good friend, and homemaker. She was known and respected by many in her community for her giving nature, wisdom, and efficiency in getting things done. If you were having trouble getting something passed by city hall, a visit to Pat was the solution.

Lately, however, Patricia felt trapped by her reputation. Her mother had been ill and was requiring extra time, and her daughter wanted to move back home to "rethink" her career choice. Although she had backed off several committees, she was finding it increasingly difficult not to lash out—in a decidedly "unPatrician" way—when meetings lasted too long or someone was determined to grandstand some trivial point. She had even begun to resent calls from friends. They no longer seemed refreshing respites but had become intrusions. She felt inexplicably angry much of the time.

Thirty percent of menopausal women find themselves struggling with psychological symptoms that include depression, anxiety, and irritability.[6] Fluctuating hormones make one's mood seem out of control and volatile. Little and big things and sometimes "nothing" lead to feelings of anger. Other women complain of a sense of being flat and emotionless. All such reactions can be precursors to depression.

I've Never Felt This Way Before

Colette is depressed. Her changeable moods have almost gotten her fired and necessitated a reprioritizing of her job, a humiliating and uncharacteristic event. Her attempts to cover memory lapses have resulted in her stress nearing panic proportions. She has begun to double and triple check her work, making her appear even more out of control.

At home she has no sexual interest in the husband she has loved dearly for twenty-five years. She feels ugly and fat. If her income weren't needed to help her grown daughter finish school and for her mother's care, she would go to bed and stay there. Lately she has been having dizzy spells, which her doctor assures her are nothing to worry about—but she does. This didn't happen overnight. The emotional and psychological changes she is experiencing at midlife tend to creep up rather than pounce. Often it takes a while to fully acknowledge that something is different and no improvement is in sight.

Colette has plenty of reason to feel upset, depressed, and stressed. Her whole life feels unfamiliar—out of sync and off balance. She worries she is losing her mind and fears she will never feel "normal" again. The amalgam of hormones, societal attitudes, and personal circumstances combine to make this a challenging time for her—but one that will end. Currently Colette does not view menopause as an "opportunity" to review, renew, and revamp, but as her symptoms subside, she will, and new fulfilling patterns of living will emerge.

When I was a child, I rarely finished a school year in the same school. My father's job required many moves. Somehow I discovered a wonderful advantage of frequent relocation. As the perpetual "new kid," I had the opportunity to repeatedly start over. I could be outgoing or quiet. I could shed aspects of my personality that didn't fit or had become burdensome.

Menopause is similar. The misery that sometimes accompanies it provides motivation to reevaluate. It is an opportunity. Feeling out of sorts gives impetus to doing things differently. Few people redefine themselves unless and until staying the same becomes too painful. The teenager emerges from puberty empowered and moving toward an integrated adult personality. The menopausal woman emerges empowered and ready for the next stage of life. There, the lessons of a lifetime provide richness to her own life and sustenance for those she influences and loves.

I'M TOO DEPRESSED TO MAKE CHANGES

Problems with depression occur more frequently during the perimenopause than during the postmenopause, when hormone losses have evened out. Suggestions for overcoming depression are poorly received. Starting something new or simply returning to healthful patterns seem almost impossible for a depressed woman. However, healthful interventions do work, even if they are initiated slowly and begun with a poor attitude. With depression, the expression "just do it" finally makes sense.

For the curious . . . The duration of untreated depression is six to nine months with a 50 percent chance of recurrence.

Depression in menopause is more likely to occur if a woman has been depressed in the past and has a family history of depression. In contrast to conventional wisdom, it is not women mourning the loss of their youth who are at greatest risk for "the blues" but women in their thirties who are married and have young children. During midlife depression, or any depression for that matter, medical complaints, like sensitivity to pain and cardiovascular and gastrointestinal problems, increase. Sleep problems are common.

The seriousness of a depression depends on its duration, severity, and number of symptoms. Sometimes there are no overt signs of depression except for a lack of energy. In other cases depression presents itself with a lack of capacity to enjoy previously pleasurable things or an inability to shake a negative frame of mind (dysphoria). Since concentration and memory are negatively affected, functioning is less than optimal. Feelings of self-loathing or poor body image are common. Negative attitudes toward life, anxiety, and an agitated sense of anticipation, dread, or fear can occur before, accompany, or be the aftermath of depression.

Major depression interferes with work, sleep, appetite, sex, and enjoying relationships and it lasts more than two weeks. It may be accompanied by thoughts of suicide and delusions or hallucinations. There may be no obvious cause, or the reaction to a person's circumstances may appear out of proportion to reality. When a depressed person starts the day, life doesn't look good and it doesn't improve as it continues.

Major depressions are currently thought to have both biological and psychological components. Deficiencies in neurotrans-

110

mitters such as norepinephrine and serotonin in brain cells of the limbic system and hypothalamus and newly discovered roles for steroid hormones (adrenal corticosteroids and estrogens) are known to affect mood, as is progesterone.[7] Such hormonal connections undoubtedly contribute to the fact that depression is twice as common in women as in men.

GETTING OUT OF A BLUE FUNK: THIRTEEN THINGS YOU CAN DO

Determining the exact hormonal component of depression, while taking into consideration the normal stresses of menopause, is not always easy. Studies have found a clear peak in psychological symptoms and insomnia in women, but not in men, between the ages of forty-five and fifty. This precedes, by five years, the peak incidence of hot flashes and sweats.[8] The fact that many women experience relief when given hormones is an obvious confirmation of a hormonal link. When it comes to midlife malaise, hormonal changes clearly offer an explanation apart from the fear of growing old, empty nests, and societal expectations. Feeling "crummy" is real and is caused by a variety of factors that need to be evaluated. Here are some ideas about what to do:

1. Join a support group. In most every aspect of life, talking things over with others provides insight, knowledge, and the comfort of knowing you are not the only person feeling the way you do. Women in different stages of the menopausal journey can provide practical suggestions, while assuring one another that this is indeed a passage, not an end point. Reassurance can confirm that the destination offers hope for the future. Menopause support groups are available in most communities and at women's health centers or can be started by a number of like-minded women.

For the curious . . . Depression can actually cause an escalation of bone loss either because of excess cortisol and/or because one tends to be less physically active.

2. Go see a qualified counselor. Sometimes an objective stranger is just the ticket to help put your life in perspective. A professional can affirm your direction and decisions, provide a sounding board, and provide insight and understanding into your behavior and emotions.

3. Exercise is always the miracle tonic for what ails you. This is so even if all you can muster is taking the stairs instead of the elevator. Exercise has both psychosocial and biological benefits.[9] It impacts serotonin regulation and enhances chemicals that affect mood (synaptic dopamine, catecholamine, opiates). The most dramatic impact of exercise is seen among women who have not been exercising. Their choice of exercise is not as important as the fact that they are doing something. Consistency is vital.

4. Pay attention to what you eat. Your mood is linked to what goes in your mouth. To relay nerve impulses, the forty-odd neurotransmitters needed for brain function must have nourishment. Low levels of serotonin can cause irritability, aggression, insomnia, depression, and powerful carbohydrate cravings. High levels lead to calmness, better sleep, even drowsiness. Carbohydrates boost serotonin levels. Protein increases dopamine and norepinephrine, which improves mental acuity, overall mood, and the ability to cope with stress. Get natural mood enhancers going early—do not skip breakfast.

Limited use of caffeine energizes some people and improves concentration but exacerbates symptoms in others. Sugar causes depression in some people. Chocolate, despite the sugar, is a mood elevator because it increases serotonin levels, gives a blast of caffeine, and increases phenylethylamine, a chemical responsible for a euphoric feeling somewhat akin to love. Besides, it tastes good.

For the curious . . . Women are more likely than men to drink heavily when depressed.

5. Try supplements. Falling estrogen levels and hormonal imbalance can affect the levels of calcium and magnesium in the body. The result can be nervousness, anxiety, loss of a sense of well-being, and depres-

112

sion. Folic acid, which works best with adequate B12 levels, helps the body manufacture and use estrogen and form healthy red blood cells, while excess use (over 400 micrograms) can cause gastrointestinal side effects, sleep difficulties with vivid dreams, lethargy, and irritability.

Hormone replacement therapy may cause deficiencies in both folic acid and certain B vitamins. B6 deficiency is linked to depression, fatigue, insomnia, and loss of libido. B vitamins are also important in conversion of your food into energy and the production of serotonin. Caffeine, alcohol, sugar, aluminum, soda drinks, antacids, antibiotics, and diuretics can contribute to excess excretion of vitamins.

6. Try herbs. Saint-John's-wort has few side effects and studies in Europe indicate its effectiveness for short-term use (six weeks or less) for irritability and anxiety of menopause. It has been billed as "the natural Prozac." It is not the choice for serious depression but can be effective for mild to moderate forms. Saint-John's-wort can increase the body's sensitivity to the sun.

Hops, passion flower, skullcap, chamomile, and valerian can be taken in capsule or tablet form or in alcohol-free tinctures or made into teas. Ginkgo is recommended (80 milligrams three times a day) if you are over fifty.

Garum armoricum is not an herb but a deep-water fish found off the coast of Brittany and sold in capsule form as Stabilium. It has been reported to be a safe and effective nutrient for reducing anxiety in healthy people in a number of studies.

7. Check the weather. Seasonal blues may have a genetic component and can exacerbate depression and feelings of sadness. If you tend to overeat, sleep more, and feel sad during winter months, you may need to look into the effect lack of light has on your moods. Consider light therapy if this is a problem for you.

8. Look inward. Write down the stresses you are dealing with and consider how you can modify your lifestyle to make your life more healthful and satisfying. Learn to journal. Learn to pray. Be quiet for at least thirty minutes a day. Practice doing nothing. Discover silence, prayer, and meditation.

9. Take up a hobby or activity you have neglected or always wanted to do and block time for it on your calendar.

10. Do something for others—unless you are a lifelong codependent always doing something for others and never attending to your own needs!

11. Check for other medical conditions. Diseases that produce signs traditionally thought to be menopausal are often overlooked at midlife. Thyroid and adrenal problems have a direct effect on mood (see chapter 20).

12. Try hormones. The choice of hormones for moods is a personal one, but hormones can make a significant difference in moods, for better *and* for worse (see chapter 17 for more information).

13. Try medication. Severe and lasting depression (over six months) can change the biochemistry of the brain to a point that

For the curious . . .

Estrogen alters the concentrations and availability of neurotransmitter amines, including serotonin. It increases the rate of degradation of monamine oxidase, the enzyme that breaks down serotonin. It displaces tryptophan from its binding sites, which allows it to be available to the brain where it can be metabolized to serotonin, and enhances its transport. Progesterones increase monoamine oxidase activity thereby reducing levels of brain serotonin.

After a hysterectomy in which the ovaries are also removed, the hormonal effect on mood is very evident. Depression and feelings of sadness or being blue are very common. A number of studies have shown psychological stress to be relieved by hormone replacement.[10] While estrogen replacement improves mood in healthy women, it is not the treatment of choice for those severely depressed. There is some evidence that estrogen may protect against depression in older women.[11]

medication is needed. This does not mean that psychological insight, exercise, and other interventions are not necessary.

- Tricyclic antidepressants: Norpramin, Pamelor, etc. These are a first line for moderate to severe depression because they work well and are easy to monitor in blood levels to determine correct dosage.
- Selective serotonin reuptake inhibitors: Prozac, Zoloft, Paxil, etc. These are for major depression and have fewer side effects than some of the older versions. Blood levels should be monitored to ensure adequate dosing and to evaluate side effects, such as becoming manic. They usually take two to three weeks to begin to have an effect.

Pearls of wisdom for keeping your spirits up . . .

1. Women who are prone to depression are more likely to be depressed during menopause.
2. Feeling "out of sorts" can be a prime motivator for making necessary changes.
3. Exercise is cheaper than therapy.

10

Sex and Headaches

It's true. Sex can be a headache at any time of life. It's also true that a headache is the proverbial excuse for not participating. However, sex and headaches, for our purposes, are linked only in their tendency to cause problems during menopause.

MY SEX LIFE IS DEPRESSING!

Dan slammed the door behind him so hard the picture rattled momentarily on the bedroom wall. Louise pulled the covers up around her neck, fluffed her pillow, and made an effort to act like sleep would follow. As sounds from the TV wafted into the room, she stared at the clock, debating whether to get up and try again to explain to Dan that her lack of sexual responsiveness was not a measure of his lovemaking ability, nor did it reflect a change in her feelings for him. This was not their first argument over sex, and she knew more were forthcoming, but she was so tired of trying to explain. How could she tell him what was wrong when *she* didn't even know?

Eventually this combination of crisis and chemistry would offer Louise an opportunity to face her sexuality with greater honesty and courage than she had managed to muster at any other time in her life.

Not all perimenopausal and menopausal women experience changes in their sexual patterns, but enough do to justify making it part of a survey completed in 1994 by the North American Menopause Society and the Gallup organization. They asked menopausal women if they had experienced sexual changes, and if so, what those changes were.[1] Here are the results:

Decreased interest in sex—62 percent
Vaginal dryness—55 percent
Depression and sadness—44 percent
Anxiety—33 percent
Feeling unattractive—33 percent
Painful intercourse—32 percent

When pollsters asked women in general, aged forty-five to sixty, who were in menopause or postmenopausal or who had had a hysterectomy, if their sex lives had changed, 55 percent of women said no. Seven percent said it had increased. And 30 percent said it had decreased. Half of the women who said their sexual activity had changed reported it had decreased in frequency, while 36 percent of this "yes it has changed" group felt the frequency was the same.

It's interesting that while actual behavior remained close to the same, attitudes changed. Menopausal women reported feeling satisfied sexually even when they experienced less arousal. Louise had tried to explain this to Dan, but it was hard for him to understand. This finding was reflected in the Massachusetts Women's Health Study II. Being postmenopausal affected desire, attitude, interest, and arousal, but frequency and satisfaction remained the same. When frequency was decreased, it had as much to do with the availability and relationship with a partner as with anything else.

Older women were found to use less fantasy, foreplay, and oral sex in their lovemaking. As Louise discovered, physical discomfort plays a role in sexual satisfaction. The effect of less estrogen on vaginal tissue causes complaints of vaginal dryness, painful intercourse, difficulty reaching orgasm, and vaginal tightness. Even when a woman feels very aroused, the normal weeping of fluid from the vaginal walls that makes intercourse comfortable is absent or diminished.

Menopause affects desire, perceptions, and attitudes about sex, but so does marital status, recent surgery, psychosocial symptoms, smoking, and the woman's partner. When surveyed, menopausal women generally agreed they had less interest in sex as they aged. They also reported that satisfaction was positively related to self-assessed health, marital status, and partner characteristics. *The 1996 Wyeth-Ayerst Fourth Annual Menopause Report* of 1,300 women and 1,000 men (between the ages of forty-five and sixty-five) found that more than 90 percent of those married or with partners were sexually active and found their sexuality to be fulfilling and enhancing.

Louise and Dan can take heart in the fact that their sex life will most likely improve once Louise passes through the perimenopause and her hormone fluctuations are reduced. They may even find sex better than ever if they seize this time of crisis to honestly assess their sexual relationship. They should use this opportunity to examine their relationship in light of their shared experiences, their heretofore unfaced truths and responsibilities, and the mutual desire to measure their experience by the intimacy it generates instead of the orgasm. Their response might very well be, "Why didn't we do this before?"

FEELING SEXY ISN'T EASY

Forget what it looks like in the movies! Being able to respond sexually is physiologically and psychologically complex. Responsiveness involves several phases (excitement, plateau, orgasm, and resolution). One aspect may be affected by hormones and another may not.[2] In fact there is great variation from person to person in how hormones affect one's ability and desire to respond sexually. One of the arguments against castration for pedophiles is that there are some people who are still capable of sexual function even when hormone levels are severely reduced.

Clearly, sexuality is dependent on much more than hormones, or any one hormone. Biochemically, interest in sex is probably due to a combination effect of hormones. When interest wanes, a reduction in growth hormone, DHEA, decreases in glucose tolerance, "adrenopause," and lower levels of sex hormones are probably all involved.[3] Women who make love more frequently have been observed to have higher levels of DHEA and androstenedione, the major androgen—the hormone that affects sex—of menopause.[4] Even the thyroid gland affects sex by lowering the energy level. Excess prolactin from the pituitary gland diminishes sexual arousal and desire.

HORMONES: CAN THEY BRING BACK THAT LOVIN' FEELING?

Whether estrogen increases libido directly is simply not known, although there are no reports of it lessening desire. A few studies of estrogen use show improvement in desire, enjoyment, and orgasmic frequency, as well as overall improvement in mood. However, such benefits may be secondary.[5] Certainly better vaginal health, attained from the use of estrogen replacement, reduces pain and discomfort. In general, just feeling better will make sex more satisfactory. It is also worth noting that progesterone, for a small group of women, tends to diminish sexual interest.[6]

When it comes to sex, you should consider hormonal therapy as one piece of the puzzle that also includes many physical and social factors. Hormone losses tend to occur when there are other problems and pressures in a woman's life. The answer to sexual responsiveness lies within the big picture, rather than the snapshot of hormones.

TESTOSTERONE: IF IT WORKS FOR MEN, I'LL TRY IT!

There is a 28 percent drop in the production of testosterone by the ovaries at menopause, yet the ovary still accounts for 40 percent of the testosterone produced by menopausal women (see chapters 17 and 20). As with all hormones, just adding more is not always the answer. Androgens, the "traditional" male hormones, have been used in hormone replacement since the fifties. For some women, androgens increase sexual desire, fantasies, and arousal. There are few good studies, because baseline orgasmic frequency and enjoyment are not automatically linked to increased desire and arousal. In other words, some people respond despite poor attitudes.

Compared to the loss of estrogen at menopause, the loss of testosterone is not as dramatic. While helpful for some, its addition has, in the past, been plagued with side effects, such as increased facial hair, acne, clitoral enlargement, and hoarseness. There is also concern that lipid panel changes caused by androgens could increase the risk of heart attack. The newest version of androgen therapy, Estratest, eliminates most of these problems. Studies indicate that about 33–45 percent of women who take Estratest report improved sexual functioning.

SO WHAT'S THE ANSWER?

While sexual desire and response is a complex issue, two common mind-sets tend to make sexual expression more difficult for women. They are:

1. the inability to accept ourselves as the unique sexual persons we are
2. our reluctance to admit that we are in control of how we experience our sexuality

The vast majority of women are capable of responding to sexual arousal. Even in this day and age, however, some women refuse to familiarize themselves with their own sexual anatomy. For others, it isn't ignorance of how things work that is the problem, but failure to examine the personal values we hold from our culture or religion. The truth is there has always been a connection between our sexuality and our spirituality. Accepting that we are the unique sexual persons we are involves a concerted effort to examine, educate, and explore.

Accepting the fact that we have control over our sexual responses implies that we are in charge of how we experience our sexuality. How we interpret what is happening in our body is determined by our mind. Enjoying a sensory experience requires an opening of body, mind, and soul—essential ingredients to fully immersing oneself in a sexual moment.

Here are some ideas to try when sex isn't all it is supposed to be.

1. Be open to breaking old patterns. Reprioritizing life should not stop with careers, hobbies, and relationships. Sex also needs to be reevaluated for patterns and habits that no longer work. Adapt to your body—when do you feel most like sex? If your answer is never, pay closer attention and keep track of the fleeting thoughts that go through your mind and when they occur—daily, weekly, cyclically. Write them down along with what you did about them.

2. Broaden your concept of what is sexual. Don't equate sex with vaginal intercourse only. Pleasure is possible through touch, holding, and just being close. Since you are the world's authority on what pleases you—discover yourself. If you aren't comfortable with yourself, how can you possibly be comfortable with someone else? Don't deny yourself new ways to feel alive and satisfied because you've never questioned your sexual routines.

3. Take advantage of the fact that midlife men are getting older too. For the first time, the man in your life may be open to something other than "Wham, bam, thank you, Ma'am" sex. Changes in midlife men cause changes in appetites and in the meaning they give to sex, and you may find yourself closer to the man in your life than at any other time of your relationship. As the menopause sex survey indicated, satisfactory sex is highly dependent on the type of relationship a woman has with her partner. Love, the great aphrodisiac, has more to do with pleasure than hormones do.

Think about it . . . Have you ever taken the time to look at your genitals? Use a mirror and discover the entire area. Which areas are most sensitive to your touch? If you have trouble doing this exercise, try it several times until it becomes comfortable. Can you see your genitals like an artist might—as a beautiful flower?

121

4. Throw out outdated ideas about sex and aging. Long-term relationships don't have to be boring. Richness comes with familiarity and shared history. New midlife loves can trust in the ability of ripened personalities no longer feeling the need for game playing. What a refreshing act—being able to ask for what you really want! Neither the act of sex nor its pleasure is an entitlement solely of the young.

5. Always use a vaginal lubricant (see chapter 5).

6. Allow yourself sexual thoughts. Daydream a little and/or call your partner during the day. In your mind's eye, see yourself enjoying a romantic interlude.

7. Don't play catch-up when you enter the bedroom. If you are already thinking sexually, you can become easily aroused. If you haven't been thinking about sex, it will take time to focus and be aroused. Just as a teakettle that is on simmer needs little heat to get it boiling, so will you. Think of a satisfying past experience or what you would enjoy doing—some people enjoy daydreams acted out with a trusted partner. Focusing on strong sexual thoughts can help block out negative thoughts and performance fears.

8. Allow yourself to play. Where is it written that sex is work? When we worry over every detail, we make sex laborious. Leave troubles, anger, and insecurities outside the bedroom and just play. If it is fun and helps you share pleasure, incorporate adult toys and play dress up or down.

9. Allow yourself to experiment. Most people are not easily orgasmic in every position. To find what works for you, have fun rearranging legs and body parts. In contrast to conventional wisdom, the vagina is not passive. Show off the results of your Kegel exercises by tensing and relaxing vaginal muscles and both you and your partner will benefit.

10. Make sure you feel aroused before intercourse. You may need more touching and stroking than in the past. The good news is that your partner probably does too. Take your time and let natural body responses prepare you physically, while you focus on the sensations—not on how you are doing. Stop if you need to, relax, talk, and begin again. With sex, you can practice until you get it right!

Think about it . . .
Seven ways to improve your body image:
    Look at what is not working in your life.
      (Diets?)
    Stop self-talk that undermines. (For example,
      my thighs are huge!)
    Stop comparing.
    Get realistic.
    Mourn what needs to be mourned.
    Feel strongly about something outside
      yourself.
    Examine the standard by which you measure
      self-worth.

11. Feel better about your body. Your body does not solely define what makes you unique and lovable. Besides who you are as a *body* person, you are also a *social* person who is loved and respected because of the way you treat and interact with others. You are an *achieving* person who has a lifetime of affirmations, accomplishments, graduations, and personal successes. Finally, you are a *spiritual* person whose beliefs and values define life and supply reason and strength to carry on. Remembering you are more than any one part—and even more than the sum of your parts—improves self-image.

If your body is not what you would like it to be, recall the totality and complexity of who you are. Men do this all the time, which is why they don't worry about a few extra pounds. They remind themselves they are good coaches, adequate providers, dependable lovers, and attentive fathers. Do you see yourself in only one dimension?

Combat negative thoughts by focusing on your positive features and paying attention to exactly how and when you put yourself down. When you understand when you are most vulnerable and how you undermine yourself, you can bypass your put-down cycle by substituting more positive statements.

12. Don't claim to have a headache unless you really do. If you don't want to have sex, don't. But practice saying no honestly so you can say yes honestly and enjoy the experience.

13. If you are experiencing antidepressant-induced sexual dysfunction, recent research has found *Ginkgo biloba* to effectively restore function in at least 84 percent of the people affected.[7]

A HEADACHE IS A HEADACHE IS A HEADACHE, EXCEPT WHEN IT'S A MIGRAINE

When Melissa told her husband she had a headache, it was definitely not an excuse for avoiding sex. In fact migraines were what announced to her that she was entering the perimenopause. Headaches, particularly migraines, occur more frequently in women and have traditionally been dismissed as evidence of a woman's volatility.

For the curious . . . Migraines are three times more common in women than in men. Seventy percent report onset prior to menses but a second onset is common from ages thirty-five to fifty.

Overlooking hormones as an important factor related to migraines' etiology, timing, and severity is not smart. Changes in estrogen levels during menarche, menstruation, birth control use, pregnancy, and menopause are related to and cause shifts in the pattern and frequency of headaches. While many women find relief as estrogen levels are lowered at midlife, others, like Melissa, begin to suffer headaches for the first time during the perimenopause. The pain they feel results from dilation and distention of the blood vessels between the scalp and the skull.

A migraine may occur with or without an aura, a visual image of light or color, or a blind spot that disappears within twenty to thirty minutes after the headache begins. It is believed that a person who has a family history of migraines may have a lowered response threshold to external triggers and internal hormonal changes that in turn activate the migraine sequence. Migraines are different from other headaches because they cause more diffuse and severe head pain, more severe vomiting, are likely to last several days, and are usually one-sided.

Migraine "triggers" can vary greatly. Melissa did not realize it, but her afternoon snack of chocolate, her high-stress lifestyle, and her changing hormonal patterns were all culprits. Other people react to humidity, changes in altitude or barometric pressure, flashing lights, loud noises, histamine, stress, and certain foods besides chocolate, like dairy products and those containing MSG, nitrites, sulfites, or tyramine (found in ripe cheese, lima and pinto beans, raisins, organ meats, beer and wine, etc.). Alcohol can also trigger headaches.

Tension headaches can also increase at midlife. A woman may have several types of headaches, and rarely are they a sign of serious disease. You should see a doctor, however, if their pattern changes acutely, they get progressively worse, or changes in vision occur.

A "rebound" headache occurs when medication taken to alleviate pain actually causes headaches, necessitating a weaning-off period. Keeping a daily diary is helpful in determining what may contribute to your headaches. You may discover, for example, that a glass of wine triggers headaches only when consumed just before a period or when your Aunt Emma comes for a visit. Frequently two or three things plus your hormonal status combine to make a difference at one time and not another.

Since food allergies are notorious for causing headaches, a three-week elimination diet (a physician specializing in allergies can provide a list of what to eliminate) will help you pinpoint foods you are sensitive to. Reintroducing dairy, gluten, and other foods into your diet after not eating them is a dramatic way to discover allergic reactions and perhaps the source of your pain. Once you become aware of headache triggers and their unique timing, you may be able to eliminate or reduce the headaches. You can do this by carefully monitoring your lifestyle and habits.

125

WHAT CAN I DO ABOUT MY HEADACHES?

There are a number of ways you can treat your headaches. Some will be of help to one person, some to another. But there are many success stories related to these suggestions.

1. Try herbs. Since headaches can have a variety of causes, it is difficult to recommend just one herb. However, using herbs in a relaxing bath can be soothing, particularly for stress headaches. Belladonna, taken orally, helps some people when headaches are severe and come on suddenly. Chamomile is also recommended. Feverfew *(Tanacetum porthenium)* has good documentation for migraines.[8]

2. Try Depakote *(divalproex sodium).* It reduces headache episodes among half of its users. Keep up to date with other new products. In the last several years a number of medicines have been developed that bring rapid relief from acute migraines. Several new drugs are being tested and will be available soon.

- Sumatriptan (Imitrex) acts selectively on serotonin mechanisms and helps stop and prevent migraine attacks. For most women, it works well with few side effects. It is now available in both oral and injectable forms and within a short time will be available as a nasal spray. Anyone with cardiovascular disease needs a doctor's advice about the wisdom of using Imitrex.
- Prozac and Paxil are not approved by the FDA for migraine, but some people have found relief with fewer side effects than with some of the older antidepressants.
- Beta-blockers such as Inderal may be effective but may produce depression, lethargy, fatigue, weight gain, and impaired insulin secretion.

3. Consider conventional standbys such as the following:

- *NSAIDS* (nonsteroidal anti-inflammatory drugs—Anaprox, Motrin, Aleve). These may help if taken regularly once the pain begins but they can have gastrointestinal and renal side effects and may cause dizziness—the cure may ultimately be worse than the headache.

- *Aspirin* (1 gram) prevents constriction of blood vessels and gives relief if started early in the attack. Excess use may irritate the gastrointestinal tract and cause less coagulation of the blood.
- *Acetaminophen* (Tylenol) elevates the pain threshold and with caffeine acts as a vasoconstrictor. It may be used daily at whatever time your headaches are most likely to occur.
- *Diuretic* use is tricky because it can alter your electrolyte balance. Try dandelion root, a natural diuretic that does not result in potassium loss.

4. Try biofeedback (see chapter 15) and acupuncture. The effectiveness of these treatments depends largely on your commitment and regular use.

5. Eat wisely. A good diet reduces the reactive hypoglycemia (low blood sugar) and stress response that can trigger migraines. Make sure you are getting an adequate amount of essential fatty acids such as omega-3 (see chapter 13), shown to reduce the incidence and severity of headaches. High doses of B6 can cause numbness and tingling, which may be mistaken for side effects of migraine.

Avoid MSG. This food additive may no longer be found at your favorite Chinese restaurant but it is still in frozen food entrées, canned and dried soup, potato chips, prepared snacks, canned and cured luncheon meats, international foods, diet foods, weight-loss powders, most sauces, and salad dressings.

6. Try exercise, which boosts endorphins, improves circulation, and helps keep the adrenal glands responsive and healthy. While you're at it, give your neck and face a hands-on workout with a massage.

WHEN HEADACHES ARE FUELED BY ESTROGEN

If you experience frequent headaches, are you a good candidate for hormones? It depends. In some cases it helps. Some

127

women are able to eliminate the hormonal influence on headaches if they experiment with the regimen and/or method they use for hormone replacement therapy. There is controversy as to whether progesterone helps or contributes to headaches. Since scientific evidence can be interpreted either way, you have to pay close attention to what works for you. If headaches are a problem, but you want to try HRT, make sure you do the following:

- Stabilize estradiol levels. Changing estradiol levels may trigger migraines in susceptible women, so regimes that do not require an estrogen break often work best. Dividing the dose into smaller amounts taken morning and evening keeps hormone levels from fluctuating and reduces headaches.
- Change from oral to transdermal or sublingual delivery. These methods insure more continuous delivery of hormone than may be achieved with the pill form. The hormonal patch is often the best choice. This can be true even for women who wish to stabilize hormones by using a patch only a few days of the month when headaches are most likely to occur. Even among women who no longer have a period, or who have had a hysterectomy, most are aware of a cyclical pattern. Apply a patch for three days around day twenty-four to twenty-eight, when breast tenderness and bloating occur, followed by another application for three more days. This system can work well for those whose headaches are related to the cyclical drop of estradiol.
- Try androgens with your estrogen. Since response to medication is unique to each of us, some women find substituting androgens for progesterone relieves headaches (see chapter 16).

Pearls of wisdom about sex and headaches . . .

1. If sex was good before menopause, it will most likely be good again after hormones settle down.
2. Regardless of treatment, headaches that increase at menopause usually subside over time.

11

Joint Pain and Osteoporosis

Along with the obvious hot flashes, changes in mood and sleep patterns, and other typical menopausal symptoms, there are a couple of not-so-obvious ones. Oddly these two symptoms, while being less noticeable, can be among the most dangerous of all menopausal concerns. They are osteoporosis, which we will consider in this chapter, and cardiovascular disease, which we'll explore in the next chapter.

Achiness and joint and bone pain are not necessarily signs of osteoporosis. Increased pain and achiness is a common complaint of menopausal women. Although the exact connection with declining levels of estrogen and progesterone is not clear, hormone therapy provides almost immediate relief from joint pain for some women. It may be that higher levels of estrogen have an immunosuppressive effect that blocks arthritic responses.

But midlife aches and pains cannot be blamed entirely on the reduction of hormones. Often the cumulative effects of gut malabsorption and/or "leaky gut," from toxic exposure, stress, and poor nutritional practices, are at fault. (This will be discussed in detail in chapter 20.) It's difficult for people to connect aches and pains with lifestyle factors. Yet dancers, for example, are well aware that certain foods—particularly ones containing nitrates—and lack of rest cause aching joints. Thyroid problems may also be at fault. Bone pain can be a sign of calcium deficiency.

For the curious . . . Carrying too much weight puts stress on joints. A woman who is only twenty pounds overweight adds one hundred extra pounds of pressure with every step.

Even excess stress adds to muscle aches and joint pain, and stress-reduction techniques can relieve them (see chapter 15).

Sometimes the reason for aches and pains is as simple as being out of condition. As we age, we joke about stiffness as we make our way out of our favorite chair or to let the dog out at six in the morning. Lessening mobility is not a joke and it can't be dismissed as a natural part of aging. Aging is not an illness with symptoms of lack of flexibility and strength. Frailty occurs, in the absence of illness, because we fail to maintain muscle tone and strength. The addition of extra weight compounds our problems, since obesity is the most common factor associated with developing osteoarthritis.

CAN'T I JUST TAKE SOME PILLS?

These days, because of the side effects of NSAIDS (Motrin, Anaprox, Advil) and recent studies that show that relief can be obtained with less potent drugs, most physicians are recommending milder pain medications. Treatment with aspirin or Tylenol (as long as no alcohol is consumed, which combined with this medication can cause liver damage) is safer and effective when you need relief.

Think about it . . . How much stretching are you doing? Stretching not only frees muscles and joints, it strengthens muscles too. Write down all the "good" reasons why you aren't doing more exercise . . . now answer yourself.

Safer still are natural pain products, combinations of phytochemicals from the herbs turmeric and ginger, bioflavonoids, extracts of passion flower and valerian root, calcium, and vitamin C. Gamma linoleic acid (GLA), essential fatty acids, and glucosamine sulphate help the degeneration and inflammation of rheumatoid arthritis and can also provide relief for general aches and pains. You don't have to search out and measure and mix together an "anti-ache" formula; there are some responsible companies that have done that for you.

130

THREE WOMEN'S STORIES

Janine was conscientious about her health and about making her annual preventive health care checkups. She had heard about our clinic and work with perimenopausal women. At forty-one, having experienced a few fitful and sweaty nights, she decided it was time to get an overview about the menopausal journey her body would soon be taking. She was more curious than worried. After all, she had no risk factors for the real concerns of menopause, osteoporosis or heart disease. She simply wanted to know the things she might do to insure the passage would be smooth. The tests she took appeared to validate her low risk factors, and since her symptoms were minimal, the focus remained on herbal and natural methods for ensuring good midlife health. Everyone was surprised when her routine baseline bone density test revealed a loss of almost 30 percent more bone, compared to other women her age.

For the curious . . . Rheumatologists have noted that there appears to be a reverse relationship between osteoporosis (loss of bone) and osteoarthritis (inflammatory degenerative disease of the bone). You tend to get one or the other.

Katherine's test disclosed she had lost 30–40 percent of her bone density at forty-five, with none of the usual risk factors. She was shocked. A close examination of her records provided an explanation for such a rapid loss without a family history, despite good exercise habits and adequate calcium intake. Over the years her calcium had been consistently high, one indication of hyperparathyroidism, which can result in osteoporosis, and this proved to be Katherine's problem.

Eighteen-year-old Caitlin was home from college on spring break. Her mother, alarmed by her otherwise healthy daughter's complaints of fatigue and joint pain, insisted she come into the clinic. Her workup included a bone density test, which revealed Caitlin had osteoporosis. Further questioning unfolded a heretofore unknown history of bulimia alternating with anorexic patterns.

While loss of nutrients and erratic eating patterns affect the body's ability to build bone, equally important is the cessation of periods and the loss of estrogen that typically accompanies eating disorders. Adding to Caitlin's trouble was a rigorous training schedule for her college track team. Overexercise can cause periods to stop. Outwardly, none of these women were from traditional "high risk" groups, underscoring the importance of having a test to measure one's exact bone-mineral density.

For the curious . . . Of women who have hip fractures, 20 percent die within the first year and of the remaining 80 percent, one-third will be bedridden forever, one-third will never again walk without aid, and one-third will recover.

THE SILENT DISEASE

Osteoporosis is appropriately called "the silent disease." Like Janine, Katherine, and Caitlin, most people are unaware that they may be losing bone. Weakening of the bone occurs years before the most serious effects show up. In fact a person may not suspect anything until a fracture occurs, he or she develops a hunched posture, or there is a loss of height.

The general population is not the only group that overlooks the possibility of osteoporosis. Recent studies indicate that even when a hip fracture occurs, doctors and health personnel do not always think of osteoporosis. A study of nursing homes revealed rather typical results. At the time of admission, 4 percent of the patients had a diagnosis of osteoporosis, yet in actuality when tested, all suffered from it.

Osteoporosis is not just the result of our modern penchant for riding instead of walking, too much or too little calcium, or avoiding the sun. It was described in the writings of Hippocrates. It is estimated that twenty-five million Americans, mostly female, have osteoporosis. If you are fifty or older, the odds of suffering a compression fracture of the spine are one in three.[1] As painful as a compression fracture is, a hip fracture is often worse because of the loss of function and independence.

A history of hip fracture in a mother increases the risk of hip fracture by 100 percent in the daughter.[2] By age eighty, 90 percent of women and 50 percent of men will have osteoporosis if nothing is done to reverse the process.[3] In view of these statistics, there are two important facts about osteoporosis that every woman should keep in mind:

1. Osteoporosis is, in most cases, preventable.
2. It is easier to prevent than to treat.

WHAT MAKES BONES WEAK?

We have all watched dogs contentedly munch on a bone for hours without making a dent in it. Perhaps that has given us the idea that once formed, bones are forever. The truth is bones are constantly being remodeled. It is the breaking down and rebuilding of bone that keeps the skeleton youthful, vibrant, and strong. It's estimated that you are a partially new you—bone-tissue-wise—about every one hundred days, with a range of three months to two years needed to rebuild bone tissue. At least 20 percent of your skeleton is replaced every year. In fact bone is rarely idle. It is metabolically active, balancing the re-

For the curious . . .
Bone consists of an organic component of mostly collagen, which enables it to rebuild. Its mineral portion, hydroxyapatite, supplies its strength. As we age, the delicate equilibrium between bone buildup and bone breakdown is no longer as finely coordinated. Menopause is a time when bone resorption outstrips formation. Menopausal women lose about 35–40 percent of their cortical bone, the hard outer layer, and 55–60 percent of the trabecular bone, the more fragile, honeycombed inner layer. While all bones are weakened, fractures are most common in the spine, hip, and wrist. Treatment and lifestyle changes can alter this.

sorption (breakdown) and rebuilding cycles, which are under the influence of hormones (estrogen, androgen, progesterone, growth hormone, and thyroid), chemicals, or physical force. When these cycles are out of sync, bone may be broken down faster than it can be built up.

HOW DO I KNOW IF I AM AT RISK?

Bone loss is a natural process of aging. By seventy to eighty years old, women generally lose one-third to one-half of their bone mass, men slightly less: one-quarter to one-third. Genetic studies involving twins indicate risk is the result of your genes and environment. Obviously the most accurate way to know if your bone loss is accelerating and putting you at risk for fracture is to have a bone density test.

A diagnosis of osteoporosis means bone mass is reduced to the point of fracture. Osteopenia is low bone mass without any demonstrable fractures. Osteopenia occurs first, then osteoporosis. There are certain factors that may put you at higher risk than your neighbor. The following are risk factors for osteoporosis.[4]

- increasing age
- female
- white or Asian race
- early menopause
- family history
- low body weight
- small stature (petite)
- low calcium intake
- smoking
- excessive alcohol intake
- activity *and* inactivity
- high caffeine intake
- conditions that impair calcium absorption
- drug use
- taking medications, like thyroid replacement in excess, steroids, and heparin, that reduce calcium absorption

134

Be aware that alcohol decreases the levels in the body of calcium and vitamin D, elements necessary for bone remodeling. Also, a person taking 30 milligrams of prednisone daily can lose 17.5 percent of his or her bone mass in a year.[5]

Too much and too little exercise can both be risk factors. Not exercising enough is a common contributor to osteoporosis, but, as we saw with Caitlin, overexercising can be a problem when it causes periods to stop and a change in hormonal balance. Forty percent of competitive ice skaters have no menses.

Osteoporosis can occur as a result of a number of medical conditions such as hyperparathyroidism. The parathyroid hormones regulate calcium excretion by the kidneys and increase absorption of calcium in the intestines. Hyperprolactinemia, malnutrition (as in bulimia and anorexia), hyperthyroidism, rheumatoid arthritis, chronic liver or kidney disease, multiple myeloma, and leukemia, all affect calcium absorption. Women with PMS have been shown to have reduced bone mass measurements and a calcium deficient state.[6]

Older people often lack vitamin D, essential for calcium absorption, because they get out in the sunlight less. They tend to chew food poorly and have lower levels of acid in their stomachs, causing the calcium they ingest to be poorly absorbed.

For the curious . . . Osteoporosis is defined as 2.5 standard deviations below the average bone density in healthy young adults. Low bone density, known as osteopenia, is defined as 1 to 2.5 standard deviations below average bone density in healthy young adults.

FINDING OUT ONCE AND FOR ALL

Bone densitometry is the best way to measure bone mass. When risk factors alone are considered, osteoporosis is missed one-third of the time. The better your diet and exercise habits were when you were young, the stronger and more dense your bones will be as you age. Some people can lose considerable bone and remain

135

in a fracture-free zone. How dense your bones are enables your doctor to predict your likelihood of a fracture.

Measuring certain representative sites helps predict your risk for fracture of any bone. However, measuring the hip itself is a more accurate predictor of hip fracture than measuring other sites.[7] Bone loss is first detectable in trabecular bone, which is the honeycombed inner layer, and only later in the more solid cortical layer. For this reason, it is of more value to test trabecular bone, if only one site is tested. Your scores are compared to control subjects your age and to young adults. Each standard deviation from the controls means the risk of fracture increases 50 to 100 percent, depending on measurement and fracture site. One thing you cannot tell from measuring bone density is how rapidly you are losing bone mass.

A change in bone density occurs slowly over time and it may take a year or so to show major change. However, there are lab tests available that, after three months of treatment, can measure how well any intervention is working. These relatively new tests measure evidence of bone breakdown (biochemical markers) that are excreted from the body and found in the urine or blood. Such tests give information about the rate of bone remodeling that is going on right now, rather than the cumulative effect eventually seen in bone density measurements.

There are several of these new tests currently on the market. The FDA has recently approved the first blood test (Tanden-Rostase). These tests could be used to identify individuals who are rapidly losing bone and need interventions that curtail the breakdown of bone. But the urine or blood tests' greatest value lies in tracking response to therapy.

There are a number of different options for measuring bone density but the greatest precision and accuracy will be found with a dual-energy X-ray absorptiometry (DEXA) scan. DEXA releases negligible radiation, takes twelve minutes, is painless, and doesn't even require getting out of your clothes.

Standard X rays are of no value because a 30 percent loss must occur before it will be seen. Another technique, quantitative computed tomography scanning (QCT), has less accuracy but enables the technician to see a cross-sectional view of the vertebra, allowing for measurement of the trabecular bone. Vertebral fractures can occur and not cause pain. When pain is present, it is usually sudden and localized around a specific vertebrae. The area is tender, but pain can disappear after two to six weeks. Curvature of the spine (kyphosis/scoliosis) may be noted. Height loss can be an indication of osteoporosis, related to the tendency to tilt forward as we age or to disc spaces collapsing.

I WANT TO PLAY WITH MY GRANDCHILDREN

No one wants the pain and debilitation of osteoporosis, especially when it can be avoided. At midlife and later, natural loss of bone becomes more critical for the individual whose bones were weak to begin with. While we can't do much about our past, it is never too late to ensure we are currently doing what we can. We can begin by maintaining adequate calcium levels, even though calcium appears to lose some of its effectiveness in building bone during the first five critical years following menopause. It is important to understand that a well-balanced diet and an active lifestyle form the first line of defense in prevention.

THE BIG THREE: CALCIUM, EXERCISE, HORMONE REPLACEMENT

Calcium

Ninety-nine percent of the calcium in your body is used in bone, although bone is only 30 percent calcium. Calcium and exercise, even leisure-time physical activities, have been proven to protect against bone loss.[8] But ensuring healthy bones is not as easy as taking a daily calcium pill. Many complex factors enter into the body's ability to use the calcium you ingest in food or supplements. It is estimated only 25 percent of the calcium you take into your body is actually absorbed.

Calcium absorption is enhanced by vitamin D, fatty fish oils, and lactose. Vitamin D is made in the skin as a result of exposure to sunlight and most multivitamins contain the recommended daily allowance of 400 international units (IU). Sardines, salmon, butter, organ meats, and egg yolks all contain vitamin D.

Foods that interfere with calcium absorption (as well as magnesium absorption, also needed for bone growth) include those with a high saturated fat content, such as is found in red meat. Caffeine and sodas disturb the calcium/phosphorus ratio that is crucial for proper calcium metabolism. Even milk can upset the ratio (see pages 188–89).

Postmenopausal women not on estrogen are advised to take 1,500 milligrams of calcium a day, 1,000 milligrams if taking estrogen. Problems with lactose intolerance and the tendency of women to worry about their weight and reduce dairy products mean as many as three out of four women do not get adequate dietary calcium. Choosing a calcium supplement will be discussed in chapter 13.

Exercise

Besides adequate calcium, exercise is the best way to ensure strong bones. While the size of your bones is controlled by genetics, it is also true that with bone, form follows function. Bone appears to adapt to the mechanics involved in physical exercise by increasing bone mass. Remember when your leg was in a cast? When the cast was removed, you were convinced you would be known as "peg-leg" the rest of your life and that it would never look like its mate.

Reduced weight bearing from any cause results in a thinning of the trabecular (honeycombed) bone. If a muscle attached to a bone does not develop or atrophies, the bone it is attached to is weakened. By contrast, weight-bearing exercise stimulates bone formation as firm muscle increases blood flow to the area.

Unlike cardiovascular exercises that give you a clue as to how you are doing, there is no intensity of exercise that can be easily measured for osteoporosis. Obviously exercise must be adapted to the health and condition of each individual. Generally, exercise done while standing must work against gravity and is considered most beneficial. Walking, stair climbing, and volleyball build bones better than swimming or cycling, although these may be the best choice for a severely affected person.

Besides weight bearing, the benefit of an exercise is also determined by impact, that is the force that transfers from the ground to the bones of the leg, hip, and spine. A sport like tennis is able to impact the upper and lower body. Walking is still the overall choice for its many benefits and small risk. Just getting outside is healing, although exercise machines, like treadmills and ski machines, are convenient.

Hormone Replacement

Remember that the critical time of escalating bone loss is the first five years after the last period. This early and significant loss is so connected to the reduction of estrogen that it is distinguished from normal age-related bone loss. Menopausal bone loss is called Type I; bone loss that is old-age related is referred to as Type II. Type I bone loss typically occurs at a rate of 2–5 percent per year for the first five to seven years after menopause. Old-age loss, Type II, amounts to 1 percent annually. It is easy to see why women who suffer a sudden drop in estrogen after having their ovaries removed lose bone faster than those going through natural menopause and experiencing a more gradual reduction of estrogen.

Throughout most of our early life, bone remodeling is a marvelous balance of breaking down and building up bone. At menopause, the rate of bone formation remains fairly normal, while resorption, the tearing down of bone, increases. The former balance is disturbed and osteoporosis results. *Prevention of osteoporosis is a major reason that hormone replacement therapy is recommended.* The appropriateness of using hormone therapy, and estrogen specifically, will be discussed in chapter 17. Here we will highlight its effect on building bone mass.

A LITTLE GOES A LONG WAY

Anything that results in even a small percentage increase in bone mass can have a big payoff. For example, as little as a 10 percent increase in bone can reduce the risk of a fracture by 50 percent. That means that a grandmother at eighty, without estrogen therapy, has an eightfold risk of fracture. Her daughter, who has taken estrogen since menopause, has a twofold risk. Such effects are modified if estrogen is not started until later in life.

With hormone replacement, fractures are clearly reduced. When 245 long-term estrogen users and 245 matched controls, with an average age of seventy-three, were compared, the group receiving estrogen had half as many fractures of spinal and hip bones and from 15–50 percent increase in bone density.[9] Another study of continuous estrogen use showed an increase of 5 percent in vertebral bone.[10] Secondarily, estrogen prevents the degeneration of cells in the hypocampal area of the brain where the center of balance and coordination is located, preventing falls and consequent fractures.

For the curious . . . The protective effect is dependent on estrogen dose, not on how it is taken. The minimal effective dose is 0.625 milligrams per day of estradiol or estrone.

Controversy exists over whether short-term use of estrogen helps prevent fractures in the long term. Those who specialize in osteoporosis recommend beginning estrogen therapy at menopause and continuing its use.[11] However, some evidence exists that starting estrogen even in old age may be beneficial. The greatest benefit is found among those women who start early and continue long term. The protective effects of estrogen do not continue once it's stopped.

P ROBLEMS WITH T EETH M AY R ELATE TO B ONES

At first it was thought osteoporosis affected the teeth by causing bone loss in the jaw and eventual tooth loss. Now the association is considered more complex. Tooth sockets begin to deteriorate, leading to gum retraction. This pulling away from tooth surfaces leaves the non-enamel areas exposed, allowing decay, pitting, bacterial invasion, and other problems.

Think about it . . .
If you have low bone mass, ask for follow-up lab tests that include serum calcium, phosphorus, creatinine, alkaline phosphatase, highly sensitive thyroid stimulating hormone, intact parathyroid hormone rate, serum protein electrophoresis, vitamin D levels, and a twenty-four-hour urinary calcium/creatinine test. These tests will show the cause (or causes) of your particular osteoporosis.

In a number of studies the connection between estrogen and dental health has been noted. Estrogen-deficient women have more bleeding of the gums, periodontitis, and tooth loss than women receiving estrogen.[12] Deterioration of the tissue around the teeth (gingival atrophy) has been reported to disappear in response to estrogen therapy.[13]

OTHER POSSIBILITIES

While hormonal therapy has become the standard for treatment of osteoporosis in women, new approaches have been developed. A woman with risk factors for hormone use now has other choices. While none of these alternatives provide a perfect solution, they at least offer options. Some of the following have recently been approved by the FDA, while others will be shortly.

Bisphosphonates

Bisphosphonates are organic compounds that resemble the naturally occurring compound, pyrophosphate, which is produced in the body. Bisphosphonates are readily absorbed into bone, where they prevent bone from breaking down by slowing the resorption activity. This antiabsorption action increases bone density by 3–7 percent, but whether it increases the formation of new bone is not known. Preliminary studies indicate fractures are reduced by 50 percent.

The first bisphosphonate on the market was alendronate, known commercially as Fosamax; others will follow shortly. An older version, etidronate (Didronel), used for years for Paget's disease, is sometimes given at low intermittent doses for osteoporosis, but if taken continuously can worsen it. Fosamax must be taken in the morning one-half hour before any liquid or food. Three years of treatment reduces fractures by 48 percent. The long-term safety of alendronate is not known. Concern exists for the effect of its long residence time in the bone.

Calcitonin

Calcitonin is a hormone secreted by the thyroid gland. It inhibits the activity of osteoclasts so you don't have as much bone breakdown. It has a weaker effect on bone than estrogen. While it affects only the skeleton and has few side effects, it cannot withstand digestive enzymes so in the past it had to be given by injection. A nasal spray version (Miacalcin) is now available. Results of studies with the nasal version showed a reduction in bone mass loss by 81 percent, compared to the results of a placebo.[14] It has the positive side effect of lowering back pain associated with disc degeneration and fracture. Negative side effects occur in 30 percent of patients but tend to go away over time. They include anorexia, nausea, flushing, rash, and increased urination.

Sodium Fluoride

Sodium fluoride both stimulates bone formation and inhibits bone resorption. It stimulates the buildup of the honeycombed trabecular bone, but the bone produced may have less strength. It does not stimulate buildup of cortical bone. In fact some experts believe that high doses may cause porosity of cortical bone, making it weaker. Sodium fluoride simply does not work for some people, while others experience numerous side effects, such as nausea and pain. Time-released sodium fluoride is now being studied and does not appear to cause brittle bones.

Vitamin D Analogs

Calcitriol is a very potent form of vitamin D. Studies show it may stimulate absorption of calcium, but more research must be done to determine the fine balance between effective doses and those that may do harm.

Growth Hormone and Growth Factors

Growth hormones are a rich source of many substances that may ultimately prove to be important keys in building bone. In the future they may provide therapeutic options not available at the moment.

Parathyroid

Parathyroid hormone acts by preventing bone breakdown. Low doses increase trabecular bone. Too much—hyperparathyroidism—increases bone loss because calcium excreted in the urine is replaced by calcium removed from the bone.

Ipriflavone

An isoflavone derivative, ipriflavone apparently prevents bone loss and enhances bone mass particularly at the wrist and spine. Calcium-ipriflavone has been shown in the lab to act directly on bone cells, decreasing the growth of osteoclasts and thus inhibiting bone resorption. It stimulates collagen and protein compounds while binding to estrogen receptors. Its effect is somewhat like an analgesic (pain reliever). It can counteract the decline in bone mineral density in patients with hyperparathyroidism.

Pearls of wisdom about osteoporosis . . .

1. Osteoporosis is a silent disease, and without testing, you won't know you have it until a fracture occurs.

2. Calcium intake alone will not prevent osteoporosis.
3. During the first five years after your last menstrual period, there is an acceleration of bone loss.
4. If no precautions are taken, you could lose up to 25 percent of your bones during the five years following your last period.

12

Cardiovascular Problems

At first Madge Davis was sure the clutching pain in her chest was nothing. She had been gardening all weekend and every muscle in her body seemed to be protesting. However, by the time she left work, she was aware something was different from plain old sore muscles—she was having trouble breathing and the pain had now weaseled its way up her neck and into her jaw.

Normally cool and collected, Madge, a forty-eight-year-old executive, was becoming alarmed. "Ah, what the heck," she thought. "I pass a medical emergency center on the way home; I'll just pop in. They'll probably tell me I've got to cut out the spicy food."

That snap decision probably saved her life—and the fact that the medical staff took seriously the possibility she could be having a heart attack. That is not always the case.

Even cardiologists, specialists in recognizing and treating heart attacks, have been shown in studies to be three times more likely to determine a woman's chest pain is "in her head" than to conclude the same thing about a man's chest pain. Or, since most women don't believe they are at risk, they ignore or trivialize their symptoms, resulting in about a third of their heart attacks never being brought to the attention of a physician.

> For the curious . . . One in nine women aged forty-five to sixty-four has some form of cardiovascular disease, one in three after age sixty-five.

145

The conventional wisdom that suggests heart attacks are the territory of men ignores the reality that nearly half a million American women die of heart disease and strokes each year. *Cardiovascular disease is the number one killer of women in the United States.* Women are twice as likely to die after one heart attack as are men and more likely to have a second heart attack within four years after the first. According to a national survey of menopausal women conducted by the Gallup organization, only 27 percent of women aged forty-five to sixty see heart disease as a major concern and most of them don't know that estrogen replacement may reduce their risk by half.

IS IT A HEART ATTACK OR SOMETHING I ATE?

A heart attack occurs when some segment of the blood supply to the heart is disrupted. If the blockage is lengthy, the muscle cells in the area may be permanently damaged or may die. Grabbing one's chest and keeling over is a dramatic but somewhat unrealistic image of what it is commonly like to experience a heart attack. For many women the signs are anything but clear. Indigestion or bursitis may be deemed the culprit. Increasing fatigue while ascending stairs or just while doing the daily routine is far less dramatic or definitive but it may be an indicator of problems.

For the curious . . . Death from cardiovascular disease is actually more common in women than in men.

A first symptom for women is likely to be a suffocating feeling accompanied by neck and chest pain (angina pectoris). Men are more likely to have very sudden and severe pain (myocardial infarction).

Coronary artery heart disease (CAD) is the result of blood vessel disease. Heart and blood vessel diseases are known as cardiovascular diseases. Other common cardiovascular problems include stroke, cardiac arrhythmia, and high blood pressure—known as hypertension.

146

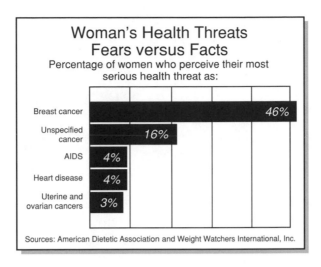

Woman's Health Threats
Fears versus Facts
Percentage of women who perceive their most serious health threat as:

Breast cancer	46%
Unspecified cancer	16%
AIDS	4%
Heart disease	4%
Uterine and ovarian cancers	3%

Sources: American Dietetic Association and Weight Watchers International, Inc.

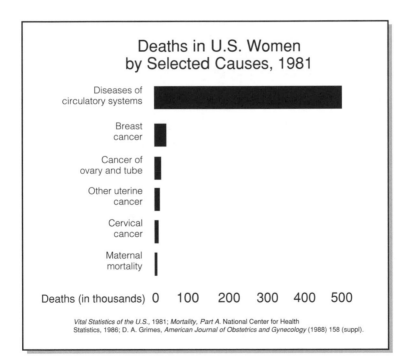

Deaths in U.S. Women
by Selected Causes, 1981

Diseases of circulatory systems	
Breast cancer	
Cancer of ovary and tube	
Other uterine cancer	
Cervical cancer	
Maternal mortality	

Deaths (in thousands) 0   100   200   300   400   500

Vital Statistics of the U.S., 1981; *Mortality, Part A.* National Center for Health Statistics, 1986; D. A. Grimes, *American Journal of Obstetrics and Gynecology* (1988) 158 (suppl).

For the curious . . . Put an aspirin under the tongue of someone having a heart attack and you increase his or her chance of survival by 40 percent.

A WOMAN'S GREATEST HEART DANGER

Fatty plaques that build up in the arteries cause a cardiovascular disease called atherosclerosis, which is the most common cause of death in women. In women aged forty to forty-five, fatty lipid deposits on the inside of arteries begin to increase rapidly. As they grow they slowly block the blood flow and may separate from the arterial wall, acting like plugs stopping the blood flow, something doctors call an "occlusion." When a major heart muscle artery is occluded, it can cause a heart attack (myocardial infarction) and sudden death. Arteriosclerosis, commonly referred to as hardening of the arteries, is frequently found in individuals

For the curious . . .
As a response to injury within an artery, smooth muscle cells multiply to try to repair the damage. Macrophages, large cells that respond to inflammation, begin to gather up excessive amounts of lipids from the bloodstream and deposit them over the affected area. Lipids appear first as yellow streaks in the inner arterial lining. Over the years "pools" of lipid build up, topped by a fibrous surface. The lesion is then called a "plaque" because it is larger and thicker than the fatty streak and rises above the inner surface of the artery. Plaques can continue to grow until they obstruct the artery or they can detach and block an artery anywhere in the body.

148

whose lipid profile reveals elevated triglycerides, low HDL, elevated cholesterol, and high LDL cholesterol.

STROKING OUT IS NOT A GOOD THING

It is rare for a woman or for her doctor to think of her as a typical stroke victim. The incidence of stroke is lower in women, because women tend to live longer than men, but over half of all strokes and 60 percent of all stroke-related deaths occur in women. One in six women will have some form of stroke during her lifetime, but they are one-third less likely to be examined for carotid artery disease. Among both men and women, hypertension remains the leading risk factor for stroke. More than 50 percent of women over age fifty-five have increased blood pressure. For this reason, stroke is becoming a serious concern.

> For the curious . . . Strokes kill more women than breast cancer.

THIS IS MAKING MY BLOOD PRESSURE GO UP!

When you have your blood pressure measured, you are calculating the amount of force needed by your heart to overcome the resistance and move blood through your arteries. It is always reported as two numbers. The upper number is the systolic pressure and is the maximum pressure produced when your heart beats. Diastolic pressure, the lower number, is the minimum pressure produced between beats when your heart is resting. Simply put, the systolic is measuring how open and supple your blood vessels are. The diastolic number measures the pressure in the arteries when the heart relaxes between beats.

Physicians are most concerned about the lower, diastolic number. A diastolic reading of 105 indicates moderate hypertension, 115 warns a stroke is likely, and 130 and above is considered life threatening. You would be considered hypertensive if your blood pressure was 140/90 or above on several occasions. High blood pressure means your heart must work extra hard to push blood through the vessels, increasing your risk of stroke or heart and kidney disease.

The American Heart Association notes that more than half of all postmenopausal women have high blood pressure. Improving one's diet, reducing salt, and exercising help lower blood pressure. Sometimes antihypertensive drugs are needed. About 27 percent of adult women, aged eighteen to seventy-two, have high blood pressure. The figure increases to about 50 percent for women who are fifty-five or over. Black women and women who smoke and/or use birth control pills are at particularly high risk.

A woman is not like a man in more ways than the obvious. Note the following less obvious differences.

- Women have atherosclerotic lesions localized in the aorta more often than men.
- Women have more incidents of unrecognized or unacknowledged heart attacks with apparently normal heart anatomy.
- Women have a higher incidence of heart attack without evidence of chest pain.
- Women who receive medication to dissolve blood clots for acute heart attacks are at greater risk for both fatal and nonfatal complications than are men.
- A treadmill test is less reliable in picking up a woman's disease.
- A woman is less likely to have her disease identified by angiography.
- Diabetes is a stronger predictor of heart disease in women than in men.
- The first recognized sign of coronary disease is more likely to be fatal in women than in men.
- Arteriosclerotic disease is more strongly predicted by hypertriglyceridemia (free fats in the blood) and low HDL levels in women than in men.

- Measured by death and poor outcome, women do not tolerate angioplasty or coronary bypass surgery as well as men.

Who is at risk for heart disease?

For the curious . . . Breast cancer affects one in nine, heart disease one in three women.

- Women who have had a hysterectomy and had their ovaries removed.
- Black women. Black women between ages thirty-five and seventy-four have a twofold greater risk of heart attack than white women.[1] From age thirty-five to age eighty-four the death rate among black women is 1.4 times that of white women.
- Women who enter menopause early.
- Women who don't exercise are two times more likely to have heart disease.
- Women with diabetes. Diabetic women are at twice the risk of heart attack as someone their age without diabetes and twice as likely to have a second heart attack. Eighty percent of diabetics die of some form of heart or blood vessel disease.
- Women who smoke.
- Women with high triglyceride levels.
- Obese women. Obesity itself is a small risk factor compared to hypertension, insulin resistance, and glucose intolerance, which often are present in the overweight woman.
- Women with a family history of heart problems, especially if her father or other male family member died, or had a stroke, or had a coronary bypass before age fifty-five; and/or her mother or other female family member died of heart complications before age sixty-five.
- Shift workers and others with social isolation and disruption of circadian rhythms.
- Women who are short.
- Women who have low estrogen.
- Women with too much homocysteine and too little folic acid.

THE LIPID CHOLESTEROL CONNECTION

Cholesterol has a bad reputation. Like the town rascal, though, it has its good points. It is vital to the hormonal, digestive, and nervous systems and is an essential part of our blood chemistry. Cholesterol is the universal building block from which cortisol, adrenaline, thyroid, testosterone, estrogen, progesterone, DHEA, and every steroid hormone known to exist is made. We couldn't live without it.

The important thing is to live with cholesterol in a balanced way. Its most important job is to carry fat in the form of lipids through blood vessels to parts of the body that need it for energy or repair, or to storage sites (frequently hips and abdomen), where it can be called on when needed. We get 20 percent of cholesterol from our diet, which when digested is sent to the liver to be processed for use. The liver itself generates 80 percent of our cholesterol.

Cholesterol becomes a bad guy when too much is in the bloodstream, piling up nasty plaques in the arteries. This causes vessels to narrow and harden, restricting blood flow and contributing to high blood pressure, heart attack, or stroke, depending on the location of the plaques. How out of balance your cholesterol is depends on many factors, such as the genes you inherited, the lifestyle you lead, whether or not you are overweight, inactive, and/or smoke.

You may have heard about one other measurement of fat in the blood—the triglyceride level. Generally, at least among women, high triglycerides are associated with higher heart attack rates and an increased risk of diabetes. Normal triglyceride ranges are 85–250, with 250–400 considered moderately high and over 400, high.

Think about it . . . If you have trouble remembering who is good and who is bad, remember L—for lethal LDL and H—for healthy HDL.

GOOD, BAD, AND THE NOT SO UGLY TRUTH: LDL AND HDL

In the liver, cholesterol joins with proteins and fat, making bundles referred to as lipoproteins or lipids. LDL is a fat bundle that contains

152

For the curious . . .
Lipoproteins come in three versions,
although two are very similar.
1. Very low-density lipoprotein (VLDL) provides transport from the liver to
unload fat throughout your body.
2. When VLDL deposits its fat, it becomes
a low-density lipoprotein (LDL), which
is the infamous "bad cholesterol"
because of its ugly habit of sticking on
artery walls.
3. High-density lipid cholesterol (HDL) is
the "good" cholesterol because it
gathers up the leftover LDL bundles
and returns them to the liver for processing, recycling, or excretion.

mostly protein, while HDL is made up primarily of cholesterol. When you eat too much fat, the HDL cannot gather up the LDL fast enough, and an increase in plaque occurs. As you can imagine, the ratio between HDL and LDL is critical. Knowing how many "good guys" to "bad guys" is as important as being aware of your total cholesterol level. Ask your doctor for a lipid profile to get all three important numbers.

WHAT CAN YOU DO TO LOWER YOUR RISK?

Just getting older increases our risk of developing heart disease, but we can't do much about that. We have little choice over our inherited risks, either. There are, however, lifestyle changes that do reduce heart disease. Below are eight things you can do to reduce your risk.

1. *Exercise.* Exercising lowers the lethal LDLs and increases the healthy HDLs. It improves circulation and increases oxygen capacity. It releases stress, which is increasingly being linked to heart attacks. Those who exercise regularly have a 45 percent lower risk of heart attack than those who do not (see chapter 14).

2. *Control your weight.* For the most effective weight control, combine a program of exercise with healthy eating and forget formal diets and diet pills (see chapter 13). Being overweight increases cardiovascular risk by more than 20 percent, and being the right weight lowers risk by 35–55 percent. Fortunately most people can help balance their cholesterol by watching their weight. Even a five- to ten-pound loss can lower cholesterol. A 1 percent decrease in cholesterol results in a 2 percent decrease in risk of heart attack.

3. *Eat nutritiously.* Please read chapter 13 carefully. Pay attention to fish oils and fiber.

4. *Try nutritional supplements and botanicals.* See chapters 13 and 16 for details. Be sure to include the following:

- a good nutritional supplement (see appendix B)
- extra vitamin C

For the curious . . .
What your cholesterol level should be:

	Desirable	Borderline	Danger
Cholesterol	200 or lower	200–239	240 or higher
HDL	55–75 or higher	35–40	35 or lower
LDL	130 or lower	130–159	160 or higher
Triglycerides	200 or lower	200–400	400 or higher

So far, cholesterol norms have been based on men. Research on women has just begun and these numbers may change for women.

- extra vitamin E
- niacin
- a combination of folate, B12 and B6
- garlic
- ginkgo
- antioxidants

5. *Take aspirin.* Taking a daily aspirin (60–325 milligrams daily) reduces the risk of heart attack by 15–25 percent. It reduces stroke risks 20 percent in men, and we assume this is true for women, until ongoing tests are complete.

6. *Stop smoking.* If you are a smoker, your heart beats faster, blood flow through your vessels is reduced, and your blood pressure increases, putting an extra strain on your heart. Smoking lowers your healthy HDL. It increases the amount of carbon monoxide in your blood and decreases the amount of usable oxygen. Smoking lowers vitamin E levels in the lungs, further reducing oxygen. Women who smoke should not take birth control pills because it increases the risk of heart attack and stroke after age 35. Even among women who use the new "low-dose" birth control pills, heavy smoking results in a great increase in heart attack.

There is good reason to quit. A smoker has more than two times the risk of having a heart attack as a non-smoking woman, more chance of dying, and a two to four times greater chance of dying suddenly. Giving up cigarettes results in a 50–70 percent lower risk of heart attack within five years of stopping, with a general readaptation of the body often in as little as two years.

For the curious . . . Forty-six percent of women's deaths are due to cardiovascular events, 23 percent to ischemic heart disease (poor blood supply eventually leading to heart attack), 4 percent to breast cancer, 2.5 percent to osteoporotic fractures, and 2 percent to genital cancer.

7. *Take cimicifuga racemosa (derived from black cohosh).* Tests with cimicifuga have demonstrated relief from symptoms of menopause with the additional

155

benefit of suppressing low-density lipids without affecting FSH secretion (see chapter 16).

8. *Reduce stress.* Not every type A superachiever develops heart disease, only those who are unable to translate the stress they face into productive outlets and/or release. Of all the emotions, anger and frustration are most often tied to heart attacks. The newest information indicates double the risk of heart attack for two hours after getting angry[2] (see chapter 15).

WHY DOCTORS LOVE ESTROGEN FOR CARDIOVASCULAR DISEASE

Young women rarely have cardiovascular diseases. Men are at greater risk than women until women enter the menopausal years, when the game of catch-up begins. Besides accounting for ten times as many deaths as those due to breast cancer, cardiovascular diseases become their leading cause of death as women age. Realizing this, physicians are often anxious (overanxious some say) to have their women patients take estrogen, since studies show that estrogen reduces a woman's risk of cardiovascular disease by 50 percent. Those who choose not to take hormone replacement therapy and follow a very rigid complementary regime that includes good diet, regular exercise, rest, and nutritional supplements will see a 23 percent decrease in heart attack and stroke.

For the curious . . . The addition of aspirin-like salicylates to foods coincides with the drop in cardiovascular disease deaths that began in the 1960s. Aspirin-like salicylates are found in products from lipstick to Earl Grey tea.

The benefit of estrogen replacement therapy on coronary arteries appears to be multifaceted. After menopause the balance between LDL and HDL changes. There is a decline in high-density lipoprotein, HDL, and an increase in low-density lipoprotein, LDL, cholesterol. Estrogen reverses these changes and enhances the clearance of very low-density lipoprotein (VLDL). Recent findings, as reported in the August 1997 *New England Journal of Medicine,* show that hormone replacement therapy may be a good alternative to cholesterol-lowering drugs. It does not affect triglycerides.

A sampling of such research includes a study of current users who have taken estrogen for more than fifteen years and have been shown to have had a 40 percent reduction in overall death rates, primarily due to significant reductions in cardiovascular and cerebrovascular disease.[3] The Harvard Nurses' Health Study (of 44,570 nurses, ages forty to sixty-five) studied women who underwent surgical menopause and took hormone replacement versus those who didn't. The study found significantly lower risk of cardiovascular disease in women who took estrogen.[4]

For the curious . . . The risk of heart attack because of sexual exertion is two in a million according to a 1996 Harvard study appearing in the American Medical Association journal.

Overall a 50 percent reduction in the rate of major coronary disease and fatal heart disease after estrogen use, with no effect on risk of stroke, was demonstrated.[5] Data from epidemiologic studies indicate that a fifty-year-old white woman has a 46 percent lifetime probability of developing cardiovascular disease and a 31 percent probability of its being her cause of death. Of the 250,000 deaths of women annually due to coronary heart disease, approximately 100,000 are considered premature.[6] Basically, most studies report a reduced risk of one-third to one-half compared to women who do not use estrogen.[7]

If estrogen prevents coronary heart disease, it is not much of a stretch to think it may prevent stroke. The closing down, occlusion, of blood vessels in the heart and brain are mediated by similar pathogenic processes. Even if stroke itself is not prevented, estrogen may still be beneficial because cardiovascular disease is the leading cause of death in stroke patients. There are fewer studies specifically on stroke. One done in Leisure World, a large Southern California retirement community, found estrogen protective. The ongoing Framingham study found a negative effect for stroke. The Nurses' Health Study found no effect. The answer should come soon when the Women's Estrogen for Stroke Trial (WEST) is completed in the next few years.

Pearls of wisdom concerning matters of the heart . . .

1. Despite your hereditary risk, you can reduce your risk of cardiovascular problems by the way you live your life.
2. Exercise is probably the single most important thing you can do to stay heart-healthy.
3. Cardiovascular problems are a major reason to consider estrogen replacement.

LATEST BREAKING NEWS

It is becoming increasingly clear that an individual can have normal lipid profiles and still be at risk for heart disease. New research focuses on tests that measure for Lipoprotein a, APOB 100, and Pattern B LDL. These significantly increase the predictive pattern for cardiovascular risks. Ask your physician for a VAP (Vertical Auto Profile) test for these lipoproteins.

Another test for cardiovascular risk is High Sensitivity C-reactive Protein. If elevated, you have a tenfold increase in risk for a heart attack. A test that measures Essential Fatty Acids (EFA) can also be important for heart health and other chronic illnesses, so have them measured as well.

The reason seemingly risk-free people still have heart attacks is because not all risk factors are known. Keep up with the research!

PART THREE

CHOOSING AN AGENDA FOR WELLNESS

If you eat well, have great genes, avoid environmental toxins, exercise regularly, and through it all keep calm and collected, you are to be congratulated. You have reduced your likelihood of many major health problems. However, you still must go through menopause.

If you haven't been so conscientious and aren't so sure what you have inherited, you still have to go through menopause. Being a woman makes it so, regardless of good or bad health habits, a great attitude, or grumbling all the way. Indeed, somewhere between the ages of forty and fifty-five, sometimes earlier, ovarian function will cease and your body must readjust to your changing hormonal patterns. Whether the transition is easy or challenging is determined by factors both in and out of your control.

In this section we will look at those things you *can* control to make the transition in and through menopause an easier one. The following three aspects of a woman's lifestyle are equally important to enhancing wellness.

Wellness Eating
- Maintain a moderate level of body fat
- Make balanced nutritional choices
- Take supplements
- Eat more soy
- Stop or limit caffeine and alcohol intake

Wellness Moving
- Exercise aerobically, for strength and for fun
- Be consistent
- Stretch for flexibility

Wellness Thinking
- Have regular checkups
- Reduce your stress
- Grow spiritually

13

Wellness Eating

Midlife compels most people to rethink the way they have been living their lives. Margo hadn't paid much attention to her health choices until her forty-seventh birthday. Her office staff gave her a surprise party with lots of goodies. The new man she was dating took her on a picnic followed by a moonlight bike ride along a local trail. It had been a fun, fulfilling, and romantic day that she would cherish.

However, getting out of bed the next morning, Margo felt like she had aged five years instead of one. "I must get back to the gym," she reminded herself as she slowly unrolled her aching body and headed for the shower. "Yep," she confirmed, "I must get back . . ." her voice trailed off as she caught a glimpse of herself in her bathroom mirror.

Margo was surprised to find that the effects of her one-day celebration did not disappear for nearly a week. That, and the discovery that Jane, her best friend at work, was going in for a breast biopsy, provided the impetus to pick up the phone and make an appointment with her doctor. To her relief, all appeared to be okay, except for her lack of exercise and the ten extra pounds that had somehow attached themselves to her. Additionally, when the doctor made her aware of symptoms she might experience with menopause, she had to admit to herself that she was probably perimenopausal.

161

Armed with the knowledge that she was in good health, but in need of some preventive measures, Margo began to look for new ways to incorporate good health routines into her day. Because her risk of heart attack and osteoporosis was moderate, and her occasional hot flashes and memory problems were still tolerable, her doctor advised focusing on good health practices that would minimize her perimenopausal signs.

Basically Margo acted to create her personal optimal health routine by focusing on wellness eating, moving, and thinking. The payoff was a delay and avoidance of the need for hormone replacement. She stabilized her weight, had more energy and fewer aches and pains, and knew she was tipping the scales against the chance of developing heart disease, osteoporosis, breast cancer, and other long-term debilitating diseases. You can do the same.

THE DETAILS ABOUT WELLNESS EATING

Mention eating, and our modern minds almost universally think dieting. Wellness eating, however, is more than weight control. It has to do with hormonal balance that leaves you energized, mentally alert, metabolically sound, and burning fat. Still, more often than not, a focus on eating and losing weight nudges out the idea of eating for wellness. In this section, we are going to suggest you can have it all—good health, vitality, and an appropriate weight.

When it was first indicated to me that food should be viewed as a drug—I rebelled. Food was love, family, and good times with friends. Today I am convinced it is also the most powerful drug you can ever consume. Firsthand experience and work with our patients have made me a believer. Incredible healing and feelings of well-being can result from relatively minor "tweaking" of the way you eat. Wellness eating is far from grim and it can be highly motivating. Doesn't sound like a diet, does it?

STEPS TO WELLNESS EATING

Among the other bits of wisdom you have acquired throughout your life is the knowledge that weight-loss diets don't work. Repeated dieting has only served to convince your body you are starving, and you can only be saved if everything you eat is converted into an emergency fat pile. The conventional wisdom maintains that starvation is the road to weight control, but that is an idea your metabolism doesn't understand. Wellness eating means eating sensibly. It simply means eating in a way that is practical, does not make you feel deprived, produces greater health, and enables you to maintain a weight that is comfortable for you, with the least amount of effort.

To simplify this even more, think about the following ten steps to wellness eating.

1. Make Changes Gradually

You can begin with the following:

- Don't shop when you are hungry.
- Plan what you will eat.
- Eat sitting down.
- Take small bites.
- Chew slowly.

2. Make Peace with Your Body

The truth is that menopause is the first time since your days as a Gerber baby when fat is in. At least some fat is okay, because the pressure is off being thin as a rail. A few fat cells keep the estrogen flowing, but too many increase your risk of heart disease and breast cancer. The trick is to preserve a weight that is healthy, easy to maintain, and possible to love.

I remember distinctly when I decided to give up dieting. If you knew me, you might be surprised to hear I had ever been on a diet. But, my thinness was only partially due to genetics. The first words out of my mouth were from my mother's exercise records. "One-two-three," I cooed. An obsession with weight was passed down from mother to child as if it had been on that fateful X chromosome.

The decision to allow myself some extra pounds at midlife was a break with lifetime attitudes. Having been challenged by a book I was writing on body image, I managed for the first time to real-

Think about it . . . What messages did you inherit about weight? Write down two commandments about weight or food from your childhood. Remember, unspoken messages are equally powerful. Have you ever questioned the validity or wisdom of what you were bequeathed? If not, do it now.

istically look at myself and at those emaciated models in the magazines. I found I liked the more "substantial" me I had become. And I saw the images on the pages of women's magazines for what they were—distortions of health and vitality. Acceptance of my body brought along with it acceptance of myself as a more "substantial" person, both intellectually and in terms of personal depth and wisdom.

A solution to your weight problem, whether it means acceptance of a few extra pounds acquired at midlife or the need to lose what has been slowly accumulating, requires a realistic assessment of where you are, the impact on your health, and your family genetic patterns. For change to be long-lasting, you need to accept yourself the way you are, quite apart from what the scales register.

Motivation for dieting, new exercise programs, liposuction, a new wardrobe, or any other change must be motivated by the desire to achieve optimal personal well-being. Changes motivated by a sense of not measuring up or founded in feelings of inadequacy inevitably fail to sustain new behavior and lead to defeat. Each slip or misstep is seen as proof of your deficiency and/or worthlessness. Inability to measure up, literally and figuratively, results in one of two actions:

1. Continual, relentless pursuit of the magic pill (the newest technique, exercise guru, diet, or plastic surgery) that will make you beautiful and, therefore, lovable, happy, rich, and worthy
2. Giving up and limiting your expectations of life, accomplishments, and relationships

Unless you accept and see purpose to your life, even achieving the societal standard of beauty will not make a difference in your feeling of being okay—acceptable and worthy of good things. This is true no matter what you look like.

Acceptance requires that you are realistic about the genes you have inherited. Drag out the family albums and be pragmatic. Forget about being a petite size four if everyone in the album has "Grandma's hips" and so do you. Strive for your "natural weight," the place where you feel good without constant maintenance and worry.

3. Always Break the Fast

Skipping meals saps energy. Breakfast is most likely to be skipped and is the worst meal to miss. Persons who study weight have learned that breakfast skippers struggle with more weight problems and lower energy levels, especially later in the day, than people who eat breakfast. Their metabolism reacts to the lack of fuel by slowing everything down. Not surprisingly, breakfast skippers also tend to snack more when they hit their afternoon lull and overeat at evening meals, worsening weight and fatigue problems. A twelve-hour fast is serious business considering the liver can only store enough glucose, the primary fuel your brain needs, for ten to twelve hours of operation.

4. Reject a Diet Mentality

- Eat when you feel hungry.
- Don't label food as good or bad.
- Don't eat it if you don't love it; if you love it, savor it.
- Don't use food to self-medicate problems.
- Eat smaller meals more often.

Just as your car won't run without fuel or runs poorly with a bad mix of fuel, your body can't function with inadequate nutrients or erratic delivery. A consistent, high-quality fuel supply in the form of frequent nutritious small meals and snacks will help keep you going. You'll note that this pattern is the opposite of what you do when dieting. The payoff is improved energy and alertness, increased metabolism, and less chance of bingeing.

165

For the curious . . . According to the National Center for Health Statistics, 25 percent of American adults were overweight (20 percent more than desirable weight) between 1960 and 1980. From 1980 to 1991, the numbers increased to 33 percent.

Limit lunch and dinner to about five hundred calories and eat an afternoon snack. Fatty meals trigger feelings of tiredness by increasing levels of chemicals that lower the fatigue threshold. High carbohydrate meals raise the level of serotonin and make you want to go to sleep. Include a moderate amount of protein to control insulin levels, maintain fuel for the brain, and trigger norepinephrine to boost energy and mood.

Snack well. Don't be afraid to eat between meals or when your body is saying it needs fuel. Make your snack a mini-meal that includes protein, carbohydrate, and fat. Avoid the temptation of settling for a highly processed sweet.

5. Drink Lots of Water

Water is a natural diuretic and appetite suppressant and it helps to burn fat.

6. Don't Eliminate the Protein

Avoidance of fat has resulted, coincidentally, in many women being deficient in their protein requirements and calcium consumption. According to a 1995 study on nutrition at Tufts University, women over age fifty-five tend to reduce protein levels to a point where they undermine their body's ability to fight off infection. Diets with too little protein result in loss of lean body mass and muscle function. You want strong muscles for many reasons, not the least being that more muscle means more calories burned. A protein shortage weakens your immune system and can even cause hair loss.

While not enough protein is a problem, so is too much. Excess can result in calcium being leached out of bones. Meats, like ham, pork, and beef, are especially high in phosphorus and can upset the ideal one-to-one phosphorus/calcium ratio necessary for calcium absorption. This can cause weak bones and muscle soreness. Avoid high protein/low carbohydrate weight-loss programs, which result in quick weight loss but modify your body's metabolism and change fat cells so that you rapidly regain any weight lost. Surplus protein can be stored as fat just like excess carbohydrate.

7. Eat Your Vegetables and Fruits

While not everyone loves to eat their "peas and carrots," there is no argument about their importance. The rule is simple—the more, the better. And the news is good. Vegetarian meals have gone far beyond the over-steamed, blanched plateful of the past. The influx of various ethnic groups into our country has brought an array of new ideas and creative cuisine.

Besides their fiber, vegetables and fruits supply vitamins and minerals, essential fatty acids, amino acids, and hundreds of special compounds that are only now being discovered. Vegetables and fruits have a decided advantage over supplements because they contain the widest mix of known and unknown health ben-

Think about it . . .
The next time you are at a restaurant, buffet, or party, pay attention to the messages you are giving yourself about food. What have you labeled "bad" or "good"? What would happen if you began to look at food as a balanced fuel you need to maintain good health, weight, and energy? What if you thought of food as a powerful drug?

efits. Their effect ranges from providing energy and protecting against disease to lowering blood pressure. The benefits of antioxidants alone—not limited to vitamins E, C, and beta-carotene but other phytonutrients (nutrients from plants) as well—come from their ability to stabilize free radicals before these highly reactive molecules cause damage. The result is less cancer and the slowing of degenerative diseases, such as heart disease. Women seem especially responsive to the nutrients in vegetables. After adjusting for all other factors, those with a high flavonoid (compounds found in plants that have a variety of healthful uses) diet are half as likely to die of heart disease as those with the lowest intake. To insure maximum benefit from your vegetables, whenever possible, select those that are fresh and organically grown. And eat a certain portion raw. We could rhapsodize forever, but the bottom line remains the same—broccoli is good for you.

8. Choose Carbohydrates Wisely

Perhaps you've seen the T-shirt blazoned with, *I've Never Met a Carbohydrate I Didn't Like*. When I was a kid, carbohydrates were called "starches" or "sugars" and categorized as "heavy" when referring to breads, pastas, potatoes, corn, processed sweets, and the like. Today the definition has broadened to include any food that ultimately breaks down and enters the bloodstream as glucose. "Heavy" or "dense" carbohydrates do so more quickly and are called high glycemic, whereas, less dense carbohydrates, including vegetables and fruit, are low glycemic because they take their time. The difference is important.

Cravings and the tendency to binge on dense or high-glycemic carbohydrates have several causes and are a common perimenopausal complaint. Being hungry for pasta, breads, cookies, and sweets can be the result of an overproduction of insulin, the job of which is to regulate the blood sugar (glucose). Ironically the problem occurs when insulin does its job too well. Eating a meal with too many *high-glycemic* foods results in an excess production of insulin and too much sugar is removed from the blood-

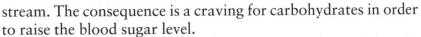

For the curious . . .
Not everyone who eats high-glycemic foods triggers too much insulin. Research reveals 25 percent of the population are not particularly affected hormonally if they decide to eat a mound of pasta or hash browns. However, another 25 percent of the population can hardly be in the same room with such dense carbohydrates without gaining weight. Most of the rest of us fall somewhere in between.[1]

stream. The consequence is a craving for carbohydrates in order to raise the blood sugar level.

You may have experienced this phenomenon when you have eaten at a Chinese restaurant: You left feeling stuffed, only to be hungry an hour later. This is so common that people often joke about it. It occurs because rice is a high-glycemic food that quickly enters the bloodstream as sugar (glucose). Insulin responds like a fireman putting out a fire, and you are left without the fuel you need to feel alert and satisfied. An obvious way to avoid an over-response of insulin is to reduce the amount of ingested high-glycemic foods. The overabundance of insulin can also be modified by adding a moderate amount of protein to your meals. Protein stimulates production of glucagon, a hormone that tells insulin to "cool it." Thus you are able to keep enough sugar circulating to avoid craving that donut, bread, or cookie.

But craving carbohydrates can also be due to a desire to improve one's mood by increasing the production of serotonin. Such self-medicating is common and explains why we crave chocolate and eat more sweets in times of stress or before a period. Low levels of serotonin have been linked to depression. Carbohydrate craving is common among the obese, those with seasonal affective disorder (SAD), and with premenstrual syndrome (PMS). Increasing PMS–like symptoms during the perimenopause can make this a real problem.

Other carbohydrate cravings are linked to poorer glycemic control either from the way the body responds to blood sugar or its decreasing sensitivity to it, regardless of how you have eaten. We know decreased responsiveness to blood sugar increases with age and is, therefore, a fairly common problem of postmenopausal women. This is due to falling levels of estrogen, which lowers pancreatic insulin secretion and decreases insulin sensitivity.[2]

Progesterone, which many menopausal women use, affects cravings directly and indirectly. In contrast to estrogen, while it increases pancreatic insulin secretion, it increases insulin resistance. This offers at least a partial explanation of why carbohydrate cravings increase during the second half of a woman's cycle when progesterone levels are highest. Secondarily, since progesterone can also heighten irritability, depression, and mood swings, it can send some women straight to the cookie jar[3] (see chapter 17).

Whatever the source of carbohydrate craving, the solution is basically the same. Maintain blood sugar levels by eating far less "dense" or high-glycemic carbohydrates than the current food pyramid suggests and balance your carbohydrates with moderate protein and fat portions.

9. Don't Count Calories—Use Your Eyes Instead

Americans continue to gain weight despite conscientious efforts to eat according to current accepted health guidelines. For the majority of Americans, something is wrong with the recommended food pyramid. Our response personally and professionally has been to endorse eating a great variety of foods, lower in calories, in moderate amounts, accompanied by lots of water. By far the largest category of food consumed should be vegetables and fruits, with protein portions based on lean body weight and activity level.

While we urge few restrictions, high-density, "heavy" carbohydrates like grains, potatoes, corn, breads, pasta, rice, and processed foods containing lots of sugar should be eaten in smaller amounts than is currently advised. Protein sources rich in arachidonic acid—egg yolks, fatty red meats, and organ meats—should be limited because after consuming them the hormonal balance of the body is changed in a way that can lead to accumulation of fat, pain, and depression of the immune system.

Proportions can be determined by a simple "eyeball" method. Your protein source provides the key. Most women, unless they are highly trained athletes, will require approximately 2–4 ounces of low-fat, high-quality protein at meals and 1 ounce more, at each of two snacks during the day—about 60–75 grams maximum. A deck of cards or the palm of your hand is approximately the size of 3 ounces of most protein sources. The "dense" carbohydrate *high-glycemic* choice (the food that quickly converts to glucose: pastas, bread, etc.) should be the same size as your protein selection. Vegetable and fruit servings are at least double the protein serving.

Eating this way not only makes fat loss easy and keeps one alert, but improves cholesterol and triglyceride levels, stabilizes blood sugar, and reduces blood insulin levels. It works because you positively influence your hormonal levels by providing your body with the food-drug combination it needs. Protein and carbohydrates, with the addition of fat, eaten in an approximate 30 percent/40 percent/30 percent ratio forces the body into a *zone* where "body and mind work together at their ultimate best," according to Dr. Barry Sears, whose books *The Zone* and *Mastering the Zone* have championed the shift away from high carbohydrate diets.[4] While researchers may debate this exact ratio and emphasize the individual nature of each person's nutritional needs, the importance of finding our individual hormonal "zone" is well accepted among those on the cutting edge of nutritional health. A balance of macronutrients is seen as essential to good health.

If eating this way sounds suspiciously like what your grandmother used to serve you, you are correct. A moderate amount of protein (never over 5 ounces at one time no matter what your requirement), lots of fruits and vegetables, and a small serving of a starch make an ideal meal. For those who like their desserts

171

and/or wine, choose them occasionally in place of the high-glycemic option during the meal. While figuring protein size is more challenging for the vegetarian, it is becoming easier as new plant-based protein products hit the stores. Tofu and isolated soybean protein powders are protein-rich without saturated fat. Unlike most diets, you are motivated to eat in a way that maintains the "zone" where you feel better, are more alert, and not hungry. Finally, laboratory blood tests confirm that the changes are from the inside out, which makes adjusting to less pasta a little easier! Your diet is hormonally correct if it enables you to lose body fat, feel good, decrease your triglyceride/HDL ratio, and reduce your fasting insulin and glycosylated hemoglobin (which measures blood sugar products in your blood). The point is that you won't have to guess if this new way of eating is good for you.

Here are some protein equivalents: $1\frac{1}{2}$ ounces of fish = 1 ounce of chicken = $1\frac{1}{2}$ ounces of ground beef = 1 large whole egg = 2 large egg whites = $\frac{1}{4}$ cup low-fat cottage cheese = 1 ounce low-fat cheddar, swiss, etc. cheese = $1\frac{1}{2}$ ounces feta cheese = 1 tablespoon protein powder = 1 ounce of seitan = 2 ounces firm tofu = 3 ounces soft tofu.

The following are rules of thumb to place you in the "zone."

- Eat regularly. Just like your car, you need a regular injection of fuel.
- Each meal or snack should contain all three macronutrients: protein, carbohydrate, fat.
- Don't count calories; use your eyes to figure proportions.
- Don't obsess over proportion. If your protein and high-glycemic carbohydrate are the correct size, it is difficult to overeat low-glycemic choices.
- Do not concern yourself with the fact that some foods, like beans, may have small amounts of protein; consider them a carbohydrate.
- Remember that whenever you eat an animal source of protein, half of your fat requirement is in your serving.
- There are a number of nutritional bars on the market and available through doctors and other health practitioners

with a 30 percent/40 percent/30 percent balance that are great for breakfast or as an afternoon or evening snack.[5]

10. Don't Be Fat Phobic

It is safe to say that many Americans fear fat. The message that fat is evil has taken. The truth is, however, fat is not all bad. It is an essential part of cell membranes, a necessary factor in digestion, a stimulus of hormone production, and it is required for absorption and movement of fat soluble vitamins (A, D, E, and K). Fat regulates how rapidly glucose is released into your bloodstream and the rate at which carbohydrates are converted and stored as fat. It is an excellent energy source. Fat is necessary for making calcium available to tissues and ensuring proper function of the adrenal and reproductive systems. Your skin, hair, and nail health also depend on fat. It makes food taste good and helps us feel full. Rather than being the source of weight gain, fat is an essential part of fat loss. More often than not it is the excess high-glycemic carbohydrates that we eat, not just fat, that are the culprit in gaining weight.[6] Our thinking needs to be refined; not *all* fat is to be avoided.

> Think about it . . . You can stop eating when you are full—if you know you can always eat when you need to.

The Primer on Fat

The main type of fat in food, stored by the body, and circulating in the blood is triglyceride. All fats have the same amount of calories. They also all have an equal ability, when in excess, to cause weight gain and degenerative diseases. High triglyceride levels in women are expressly associated with an increase in heart attacks, even when cholesterol levels are normal. It is, however, more common for people with high triglyceride levels to also have high LDL cholesterol and lower HDL cholesterol. High triglycerides are a risk factor for diabetes as well.

Triglycerides come from our liver and through our diet. Lack of exercise, high stress, and alcohol consumption increase their

173

level. The habit of skipping breakfast, eating a light lunch, and catching up with a large dinner contributes to an overabundance of triglycerides at bedtime. These triglycerides have nothing productive to do except to cause red blood cells to clump together, potentially blocking small capillaries or taking up residence at one of their favorite locations, just above the waistline.

Cholesterol is fat that moves around in the blood attached to a bubble of lipoprotein. Low-density lipoproteins (LDL) transport cholesterol to the tissues where the cholesterol only becomes "bad" when too much is available and accumulates in the blood vessel walls. High-density lipoproteins (HDL) are considered "good" because they carry excess cholesterol to the liver to be destroyed. Cholesterol is important on a cellular level during digestion. Your level of cholesterol depends on a combination of factors that reflect your diet, lifestyle, and heredity.

Sorting Out the Good from the Bad

SATURATED FATS

- mostly animal in origin
- solid at room temperature
- plant-based include liquid coconut, palm, and palm kernel

    Effect: When reduced, lower blood triglycerides and cholesterol levels and lower incidences of heart disease and cancer result.

UNSATURATED FATS

- usually liquid
- polyunsaturated (safflower, corn, soybean, fish)
- monounsaturated (olive, sesame, and canola oil, almonds, avocado)

    Effect: Monounsaturated, like olive oil, lowers LDL and increases HDL, protecting against heart disease.

ESSENTIAL FATTY ACIDS

- must come from foods or supplements

- polyunsaturated (fish oils, fish, flax, borage, black currant, and primrose oil, sunflower and pumpkin seeds)

  Effect: An essential energy source, reduces cholesterol, slows atherosclerosis, influences prostaglandin production, reduces arthritic pain, protects against heart disease, boosts immunity, and helps reduce PMS symptoms. Omega-6 (linoleic acid) or omega-3 (linolenic acid) fatty acids in primrose, flaxseed, and black currant seed oil have been found to reverse the cancer-causing effects of radiation and carcinogens.[7] Deficiency may cause swelling, increased blood clotting, breast pain, hot flashes, uterine and menstrual cramps, and constipation. Fatigue, lack of endurance, dry skin and hair, and frequent colds may also be signs of EFA shortage.

HYDROGENATED VEGETABLE OILS (TRANSFATTY ACIDS)

- used in foods that must sit on the shelf for months at a time and still maintain taste

  Effect: Margarine and other transformed fats are modified to the point they can no longer be used by the body to

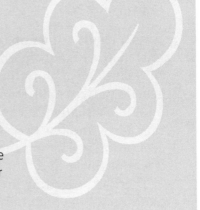

For the curious . . .
Flaxseed oil may be a particularly good protection against breast cancer in women. Barlean's Flax Seed Oil, made from 100 percent certified organic flaxseed, has been specially processed so the oil is not damaged by heat, light, and oxygen. It should be in the refrigerator of your local natural food store. Do not heat flaxseed oil; merely sprinkle it over a salad, vegetables, cereal, or spread it on bread instead of butter.

CHOOSING AN AGENDA FOR WELLNESS

make hormones and actually interfere with natural fat's ability to produce them.

DESIGNER FAT

- products designed to make foods taste rich without fat
- Olestra, Nutrasweet's Simplese, and Orlistat have FDA approval as fat substitutes; others will follow.

    Effect: Fat substitutes do not do the good things fat was meant to do; they are merely a way of making food taste rich without adding fat to the diet. Olestra prevents your body from absorbing vitamins A, D, E, K, and other nutrients. Digestive upset and diarrhea occur in at least 20 percent of people, but since digestive disturbances are common and the amount that upsets people is highly variable, many people may not make the connection between eating Olestra and feeling ill. These fats are not the way to have your cake and eat all of it!

The Final Word on Fat

1. You have nothing to gain by substituting bad fats for good.
2. Fats are an essential part of your diet.
3. Consider the kind of fat, not just the amount.
4. Remember many "reduced-fat" products are made to taste better by adding sugar.

OTHER CONCERNS ABOUT WEIGHT

As a result of menopause, chances are you will gain approximately ten pounds, perhaps even five pounds more with surgical menopause. Anything beyond that is more likely due to genetic patterns and our tendency to physically slow down at midlife. Actually your metabolism began to slow down at age thirty-five and has been decelerating at the rate of ½ to 1 percent per year. That means at age fifty it is 15 percent slower than it was at thirty-five.

There is no getting around the fact that if you want to look like you did in your youth, you must eat less and exercise more.

Even then, you still may not fit into your prom dress. A study of older long-distance runners revealed that as they got older, even they increased in girth and in the associated health risks of extra fat around the middle.[8]

Will Taking Hormones Increase My Weight?

Studies done at the University of California at San Diego compared women who had used hormone replacement continuously for at least fifteen years with those who had used it off and on and those who had never taken hormones. They found no differences in body fat distribution or composition. Participants in the Nurses' Health Study who used HRT were leaner than those who didn't, and ongoing studies indicate hormones may prevent increases in lower-body fat deposition.[9] A selection bias is possible, with the nurses in the study being aware of the health risks of too much weight and having more medical intervention. Generally the conclusion is: *Hormone replacement does not cause weight gain. Going through menopause and getting older do.*

For the curious . . . One serving of salmon or three servings of tuna or other cold water fish a week, a handful of sunflower seeds a day, or 1–3 teaspoons of flaxseed oil daily, provide enough essential oil to be beneficial.

Midlife fat gain cannot be blamed on the pill, but retaining water and feeling bloated may indeed be your unique response to the particular brand of hormone or by its delivery system. Check with your doctor and see chapter 17.

Is Being Fat Always Bad?

There is more danger of death from excessive loss or gain of weight than from simply being overweight. Whether or not your additional poundage is a problem depends on whether you are hypertensive, diabetic, or have other health concerns. The location of your fat is as important in determining the seriousness of the problem as how overweight you may be.

Why Looking like a Pear Is Better Than Looking like an Apple

Being overweight is a major risk factor if, when you take off your clothes and look in the mirror, you see an apple looking back at you—an apple shape, that is. This is in contrast to being overweight and having your fat distributed below your waist, giving you a pear shape, which may put you at less risk. Waistline size and waist-hip ratio are powerful predictors of coronary heart disease in middle-aged women. Large amounts of fat around your middle may lead to high concentrations of free fatty acids and trigger hypertriglyceremia (high triglycerides) and subsequent atherosclerosis (plaque buildup), which leads to heart disease and diabetes.[10]

GOOD THINGS TO PUT INTO OUR MOUTHS

While eating a well-balanced diet, which includes a variety of food, is the most significant thing a woman can do to influence her overall health, there are new discoveries on the horizon that can help move her toward optimal wellness.

For the curious . . . Looking like an apple is a telltale sign that your hormones are imbalanced, you produce too much insulin, and you are therefore hyperinsulinemic. It is possible to be hyperinsulinemic and not look like an apple if your triglyceride levels are over 200 and your HDL cholesterol level is less than 35.

The Joy of Soy

There is a growing list of products that are incorporating soy ingredients. For most of us, soy is a welcome addition to the American diet. Soy lowers cholesterol levels and offers protection against breast cancer for midlife women. The chief isoflavone in soy—genistein—is known to inhibit growth of cancer cells while leaving normal cells alone. The first study to show an inverse association between soy consumption and the risk of endometrial cancer was reported in 1997 by the Cancer Re-

For the curious . . .
The large study of nurses, ages forty to sixty-five, found a three to four times greater risk of heart disease for those women whose waist-to-hip–ratio measurement placed them in the upper quarter of those measured, compared to those in the lowest quarter, and a relative risk for heart disease of four- to five-fold.

To learn whether you are hyperinsulinemic, measure your waist at the smallest part, viewed from the front, and the hips at the widest part, viewed from the side. If your waist-to-hip ratio is greater than 0.80, you are at greater risk than someone who is obese with other patterns. Call your physician and follow up with an examination of carotid, abdominal, and femoral arteries.

search Center in Hawaii. In its role as an antioxidant, soy prevents cell damage and thus enhances immunity.

Dr. Lee-Jane Lu reported at the 1997 annual meeting of the American Association for Cancer Research that her study of premenopausal women who added 36 ounces of soy milk daily to their diet for a month had lowered blood levels of estradiol and progesterone (30 percent and 60 percent respectively) while maintaining normal periods. Since ovarian hormones regulate growth of breast epithelial cells, reducing these hormones could ultimately reduce the likelihood of cancer.[11] A similar study using soy protein powder was reported at the 1997 American Heart Association's annual meeting. The women in this study had less severe hot flash symptoms. A third study, reported in the *Journal of the North American Menopause Society*, found measurable and positive changes in hormonal levels after additional soy and flaxseed oil were added to menopausal women's diets for six weeks.[12] This again points out what a powerful medicine food can be.

Indeed, in countries where soy is a big part of the diet, like Japan, incidents of breast cancer (and prostate cancer in men) are far fewer than in the United States. Of course, the Japanese also eat less animal fats and more fish and vegetables than we do. They are also genetically homogeneous and tend not to be overweight and to walk more. Nevertheless the scientific reasons for why soy is a good addition to your diet are sound.

The best sources of soy are tofu, low-fat soy milk fortified with calcium, and soy protein powder. In addition to drinking soy milk, you can use it in baking or as a base for soups. Mix herbs into tofu and use it for dips and over baked potatoes. Tofu absorbs the flavor of anything that is cooked with it. Mix it with eggs, in refried beans, or in spaghetti sauce. Some find soybeans, themselves, difficult to digest but highly processed food versions can lose their nutritional value. Soy breakfast meats and cheeses (like Tofu-rella and Almond-rella) are a low-fat way to get morning protein and excellent choices for vegans who eschew dairy. If tofu isn't your favorite snack food, take heart. Massive amounts are not required to benefit from its inclusion in your diet.

For the curious . . .
Insulin's job is to take excess glucose and amino acids from the foods we eat and store them as fat. Glucagon, working in opposition to insulin, releases stored fat for use as energy. Both these hormones are made in the pancreas. Glucagon plays a part in reducing the production of cholesterol, while insulin stimulates its production. The more insulin you make, the greater the chance of too much artery-clogging cholesterol.

Green Tea (Camellia Sinensis)

Soy and good genes may not be the only explanation for lower breast cancer rates in Japan. Drinking green tea at meals—about three cups daily—may also play a part. Most important, its high polyphenol content, mainly flavonoids, makes it a powerful antioxidant with the ability to modify the body's reaction to allergens, viruses, and carcinogens. Estrogen-related cancers, like breast cancer, are particularly susceptible because of the changes it stimulates directly within the breast's estrogen receptors. Because of green tea's anti-inflammatory, antiallergenic, antiviral, and anticarcinogenic actions, you should consider drinking a cup at some of your meals. The caffeine in green tea (50–100 mg per cup) seems to have a milder effect on most people than caffeine in other teas.

Our Need for Supplements

In a perfect world there would be no need for supplements. A two-year study in the *Journal of Applied Nutrition* compared organically grown vegetables and fruits with commercially grown varieties. The organic foods had on average over 90 percent more of the twenty-two nutrients tested.[13] The type of soil, fertilizers, harvesting times, and differences in handling can make a significant difference in the nutritional value of food. It should be pointed out that in the United States we no longer use DDT because of its toxicity but we continue to be the largest distributor of it throughout the world and much of the produce from foreign countries has been sprayed with it.

Even having good food available doesn't help the individual whose lifestyle means eating on the run, grabbing processed foods, and skipping meals. Adding micronutrients at midlife to correct and counter a lifetime of poor foods and perhaps even poorer habits is a step in preventing the further development of slow-developing degenerative diseases that we may first become aware of as we age. Taking a nutritional supplement is like an insurance policy; you may never need it, but it is sure nice to have when you do need it.

181

While it is tempting in this new era of vitamin awareness to take multiple supplements, as in everything else, balance is in order. You may do more harm than good if you "load up" on something you think you may be lacking. Vitamins and minerals, like herbs, often work synergistically. In other words, they like to be in an orchestra, not solo performers. They act as triggers for important enzymatic processes, are required for repair and maintenance of tissues and bone, sometimes act as precursors to the production of hormones, while others reduce cell damage by maverick oxygen molecules known as free radicals.

Today we rarely see classic deficiency diseases. Instead, insufficiencies of vitamins and minerals are more likely to affect function and, thus, well-being. Those who are aware of the latest research consider the current recommended dietary allowance (RDA) by the government to be outdated. While the average person may benefit by following the guidelines, dosages may be quite different for people who are considerably over- or underweight. It changes for those who have chronic illnesses, especially if they are taking medications. People with digestive problems and those who are taxed physically or highly stressed may have increased requirements. Individual uniqueness accounts for a correct balance for one person versus another as do lifestyle factors such as regular alcohol use, smoking, and exposure to pesticides and pollutants.

For the curious . . . The average regular user of vitamin supplements has a college degree, earns fifty thousand dollars or more, and is likely to live in the West.[14]

Minimally, you should take:

1. a multivitamin supplement
2. vitamin E
3. calcium

There are many multivitamins/supplements on the market. Remember, the micronutrients they contain enable you to use the macronutrients (protein, carbohydrates, and fats) you consume.

They are *never* a substitute for food. Choose one that contains a variety of ingredients. Minimally, make sure your brand has vitamins A, B-complex, C, D, E, calcium, magnesium, potassium, iodine, copper, and zinc. Look particularly for a wide variety of antioxidants that help protect you from free-radical damage, believed to promote heart disease and cancer and to contribute to aging. There are many antioxidants. Don't focus on beta-carotenes alone. Foods high in beta-carotene, which include other carotenoids and antioxidants, reduce cancer. But research has not proven that removing beta-carotenes from the other vitamins and minerals they work synergistically with is beneficial. In fact it could actually be harmful especially for smokers.

For the curious . . . The Public Health Service states that four of the ten leading causes of death in the United States are associated with diet and nutrition (heart disease, cancer, strokes, diabetes), representing two-thirds of all deaths in 1991.

Look for selenium, which has recently been shown to prevent certain cancers—the first nutrient to be shown to do so in human trials.[15] And look for a variety of natural-source carotenoids, such as alpha carotene, cryptoxanthin, zeaxanthin, lutein, and lycopene. Bioflavonoids like quercetin help strengthen blood vessel walls and enhance the efficiency of vitamin C. Folic acid regulates cell division and supports the health of gums, red blood cells, the gastrointestinal tract, and the immune system. Studies also credit a deficiency of folic acid for 30 percent of coronary heart disease, blood vessel disease, and strokes. Folic acid level is proving to be as important as cholesterol level in determining risk for heart disease.[16]

Inositol aids nerve transmission and fat metabolism. Niacin helps release energy from carbohydrates and aids in the breakdown of protein and fats as well as in the formation of red blood cells. Adequate D aids calcium absorption.

Deficiencies of thiamin (B1) can result in fatigue, depression, and "pins and needles" sensations or numbness in the legs. Pyridoxine (B6) is a necessary part of over sixty enzymes and is often in short supply in menopausal women who take hormones. Its role in the manufacture of all neurotransmitters, including serotonin, means its shortage can contribute to depression. Pantothenic acid (B5) supports adrenal function and good heart health. The whole B-complex is often recommended for stress and to ensure proper energy production.

A growing number of scientific papers are calling for the same B ratio but in greater amounts than has been recommended by the RDA. Mineral balance is equally important to ensure their absorption.[17] All in all, balance outweighs amount at this stage of our knowledge, so be careful about megadoses of any one thing. After age fifty, if your periods have stopped, unless you are anemic, you do not need a supplement with iron, as this could aggravate heart conditions.

For the curious . . . Menopausal women who are not on estrogen therapy are advised to get 1,500 milligrams of calcium a day, 1,000 milligrams if on hormone replacement.

Finally, pay attention to the coating that holds your pill together. It should break down within thirty minutes for maximum absorption. Research indicates that products that dissolve more rapidly are absorbed much better than time-release products or those that dissolve slowly. Make sure that it contains none of the common allergens, such as yeast, soy, milk, egg, wheat, corn, or artificial coloring. If vitamins make you nauseous, take one with a vegetable coating.[18] There are many multivitamin/supplements on the market. For a complete list of what your supplement should minimally contain, refer to appendix B. Our workhorse at A Woman's Place is Metagenics' Intensive Care (Fem Essentials), which contains high quality ingredients designed for optimal absorption and bioavailability. Multi Nutrients (Ethical Nutrients) is also a good choice.

Extra Vitamin E

In addition to your multivitamin, take extra vitamin E, 400–800 IU a day. For a limited time, when hot flashes are a particular problem, you can increase up to 1,200 IU a day. Why extra vitamin E? There are many reasons. It is believed to be an immune enhancer particularly protective against breast cancer. Doses of 200 IU have shown significant improvement in various tests of immune strength for people sixty-five and over. [19] It is useful for relief of vaginal dryness, breast cysts, and thyroid problems. Most recently, its importance in preventing and reducing the effects of heart disease and Alzheimer's disease has made news headlines. It is believed to reduce the thickening of the carotid arterial walls and may prevent the oxidation of LDL, which contributes to the formation of plaques in arteries.

Dietary vitamin E is obtained by eating vegetable oils, nuts, seeds, green leafy vegetables, and some fruits. Too much vitamin E may cause temporary nausea, gas, or diarrhea. Persons with hypertension and diabetes should not use the oily form of vitamin E since it can reduce the need for insulin. Diabetics need to carefully monitor dosages with their physician. Vitamin E is best absorbed and utilized if the natural form (d = alpha tocopheryl) rather than the synthetic form (dl = alpha tocopheryl) is used.

For the curious . . .
Calcium is used by the central nervous system to keep nerves functioning. If the calcium supply is too low, nerves become hyper-excited and muscles go into spasm or if calcium is deficient for a long time, muscles twitch and cramp. This means calcium directly affects the muscles by affecting their contractile ability—including the heart muscle.

The Super Importance of Calcium

While 99 percent of calcium is used in bones and teeth, that leftover 1 percent floating in the bloodstream is essential for life and health. If it were missing, your muscles wouldn't contract correctly, your blood wouldn't clot, and your nerves wouldn't transport messages. Too little calcium and you are likely to suffer from insomnia, muscle cramps, and agitation or depression. You may also tire easily, experience limb numbness—and break your fingernails! Your body must get the calcium it needs from your food or it will remove it from your bones.

There are three times in your life when calcium is in extra demand:

- when you were growing
- when you were nursing
- the first five years after your last period

Think about it . . . What kinds of habits did you have as a teen? Did you drink milk? Were you active? How about your daughter or your granddaughter? Strong bone mass laid down during the teen years can help a woman get through later high-risk times.

While no one disagrees that getting the calcium you need through your diet is best, there is considerable controversy as to the benefits of calcium supplementation. The observation is made that women in more exotic locales seem to get by on far less calcium than is recommended in the United States. This does not take into account differences in genetics, diets, our relatively sedentary American lifestyle, and environmental pollutants.

No matter how careful you are to maximize your calcium intake, you will absorb only 25–30 percent of what you obtain from food or through supplements. Absorption depends on:

- the presence of other micronutrients
- the type of calcium consumed
- when the calcium is consumed
- what the calcium is consumed with

Thirteen Things That Affect Calcium Availability

1. Micronutrients
2. Caffeine and soft drinks
3. Medications
4. Amount
5. The time of day
6. Type of food consumed
7. Too much milk
8. Too much sugar
9. A high-fat diet
10. Too much protein
11. Excess insoluble fiber
12. Excess alcohol
13. A diet high in vegetables

Micronutrients. When adding a calcium supplement to your diet, purchase one that contains the following additional micronutrients to ensure maximum benefit of your calcium supplement or diet.

- magnesium—transports calcium, converts D to its active form
- phosphorus—for growth, maintenance, and repair; must be in a 1-to-1 ratio with calcium
- copper, zinc, and manganese—trace minerals that improve calcium retention[20]
- vitamin C—for synthesis of collagen proteins
- boron—for calcium balance, estrogen production, and utilization of vitamin D[21]
- silicon—promotes collagen synthesis
- vitamin B6, B12, and folic acid—for collagen production
- vitamin K—converts osteocalcin to its active form, which anchors calcium molecules within bones
- vitamin D

Caffeine and soft drinks alter the phosphorus-to-calcium ratio.

Medications. Some medications alter the absorption of calcium or may even prevent its absorption. The following may have this effect: corticosteroids, anticonvulsants, tetracycline, antacids containing aluminum, buffered aspirin, sedatives, antibiotics, steroids (arthritis), some cardiovascular medications, muscle relaxants, and antidiabetic drugs taken longer than a week.

The amount. Only 500 milligrams of calcium can be absorbed at any one time.

187

The time of day. Take calcium with breakfast if hydrochloric acid (HCL) levels are low (you are burpy and gassy after meals). Take calcium at night without food if your HCL levels are good and benefit from a reduction of night leg cramps and better sleep.

Type of food consumed. Oxalic acid in rhubarb, spinach, chard, beet greens, and parsley, as well as phytic acid found in the husks of cereal grains decrease calcium absorption. Realistically, these foods are not a major problem, considering their nutritional benefits, unless you are eating massive amounts.

Too much milk. Ironically, even milk, one of the best sources of calcium, has its detractors because excess milk can upset the

For the curious . . .

As we age, many people lose the enzyme lactase, which is necessary for breaking down lactose (milk sugar). Dairy products, like milk, cheese, and ice cream reach the colon and ferment, resulting in bloating, gas, and cramps or they may trigger excess mucous production in the nasal passages. Filipinos, Japanese, Thais, and African Americans have the highest rates of lactose intolerance.

Products that replace the missing lactase can be purchased over the counter. Some lactose-intolerant people can eat live-culture yogurt, milk products containing acidophilus, some hard, aged cheese, and goat or sheep milk or cheese. Sensitivity to sorbitol, an artificial sweetener, and fructose, found in many soft drinks, is common among lactose-intolerant individuals.

Sources of calcium for such people include calcium-fortified foods, from orange juice to soy milk, dark green leafy vegetables, hazelnuts, almonds, fish with small edible bones like salmon and sardines, and lime-processed tofu.

crucial phosphorus/calcium balance and/or neutralize hydrochloric acid.

Too much sugar depletes phosphorus.

A *high-fat diet* decreases calcium absorption in the gut.

Too much protein causes calcium leaching and imbalance of phosphorus.

Excess insoluble fiber binds calcium and carries it out of the body.

Excess alcohol inhibits liver function that ultimately inhibits absorption.

A *diet high in vegetables.* Eating vegetables aids calcium absorption. Vegetarians build bone in the same way as meat eaters when they are young—but they maintain strong bones as they age. The vitamin K that is found in leafy green vegetables and their reduced intake of animal fat and protein may be the reasons.

The Emergency Vitamin

Vitamin C is included in most multivitamins. Whether a person can benefit from additional supplementation depends on the individual. Taking large doses of vitamin C daily has not been shown to prevent colds or flu, but studies do indicate that taking extra C as soon as a cold or flu strikes is likely to shorten the course of the illness. Vitamin C can reduce the release of histamine, thereby reducing allergy symptoms. Among other benefits, it is generally believed to improve immunity, is essential in the metabolism of collagen and the manufacture of various neurotransmitters and hormones, and is the most cost-effective and beneficial of all the antioxidants. If you are deficient in vitamin C, you may suffer from bleeding gums or depression; you may bruise easily and feel tired and achy. When life's stresses begin to wear you down, vitamin C just might build you up.

Ascorbic acid is a widely used form of vitamin C that is inexpensive and effective. A few people experience diarrhea and/or gas with large doses and they may better tolerate a "buffered" C. A rebound effect (such as bleeding gums) can occur with erratic use of large doses. People with kidney problems should consult their doctor before taking vitamin C. Remember, vegetables as well as fruit are good dietary sources of vitamin C.

189

For the curious . . .

1. Having worked so closely with menopausal women, many of whom are osteopenic or have osteoporosis, our calcium recommendation has been very important and the subject of considerable review. At A Woman's Place we advise our patients to take a calcium product known as Cal Apatite or the versions for women— Fem Osteo, Fem Osteo HRT (Metagenics), and Bone Builder (Ethical Nutrients)—because of the specific formulation that includes calcium-rich microcrystalline hydroxyapatite, which is the core of all bone. It is combined with a ratio-balanced mix of magnesium, phosphorus, protein matrix, and other vital ingredients necessary for bone formation. It has been found to be instrumental in improving, stabilizing, and reversing bone loss in research studies and in our practice. We trust its preparation, which includes cryogenic processing, because of the third-party assessing to eliminate the possibility of heavy metal contamination, and the utilization of bone from New Zealand free-range cattle, raised on land where no pesticides are used.

2. Calcium carbonate has the highest amount of elemental calcium. *If it is taken properly,* it is well-absorbed. It is the most cost-effective form, but it must be taken on a full stomach to make use of the hydrochloric acid. It can cause gas or constipation. Note that some researchers consider calcium carbonate highly unusable in the body.

3. Calcium phosphate is well-absorbed, does not cause gas or constipation, can be taken anytime, but is more expensive.

4. Calcium citrate is the most easily absorbed. It has a higher cost and a lower percentage of elemental calcium and is often used in products that are "fortified" with calcium, like orange juice. Excess will not cause kidney stones.

Essential Fatty Acids

Despite our penchant for overeating hydrogenated and saturated fats, many experts claim a great number of Americans are seriously deficient in essential fatty acids. Increasingly we are asking our midlife patients to supplement essential fatty acids in their diet. Most often we recommend flaxseed oil, but high quality supplements are available for those who prefer them. They should be certified as organic in origin, extracted only by a modified expeller process with temperature not exceeding 98 degrees, and packaged in a light-resistant container with expiration date. A shortage of these oils affects a cell's ability to selectively allow materials in or out of cells and this leads to cell damage and the inability to communicate with other cells. EFAs are critical in the formation of prostaglandin, which regulates hormone synthesis. Pressure in the eye, joints, and blood vessels, and our response to pain, inflammation, and swelling are among many other vital processes that EFAs affect.

Bioflavonoids

Bioflavonoids, including proanthocyanidins, quercetin, hesperidin, rutin, flavones, and flavonols, are not essential for life, like a vitamin is, but they enhance the performance of vitamin C and thus can indirectly be very important in achieving optimal health. Research indicates bioflavonoids and C together strengthen capillaries, enhance immunity, decrease inflammatory response, and protect against diabetic cataracts better than C alone.

In combination with magnesium and vitamins B6 and E, bioflavonoids can effectively alleviate hot flashes in some menopausal women.

The best news is that bioflavonoids occur naturally with virtually no toxicity. Major sources include most citrus, apricots, grapes, plums, buckwheat, and rose hips. While orange juice contains vitamin C, in most cases the bioflavonoids have been left in the white matter of the fruit near the rind. Eating the whole fruit is more beneficial. Vitamin C in a natural product contains bioflavonoids, but its synthetic version will not, unless they are

191

added. Note also that bioflavonoids can be rendered useless by the extraction process used. Always buy supplements from companies with a good reputation that use high quality, pure ingredients and manufacture their products with integrity.

OTHER THINGS WE PUT INTO OUR MOUTHS

Caffeine

Caffeine makes hot flashes worse. It increases your triglycerides, reduces calcium absorption, and destabilizes blood sugar. Those who have given up their daily hit of tea, coffee, or sodas have discovered there is life without caffeine. Those who haven't are advised to limit caffeine choices to two a day. To be satisfied with one or two cups a day, when you have it, make it a big deal. Don't drink it on the run or out of plastic. Sit down and make it a respite, only indulging if it is a great cup of coffee, tea, or your favorite soda. Do like the English—take a midafternoon break. It is much easier to limit caffeine when you keep the standards high for enjoying it.

Alcohol

Alcohol made the government's list of *Dietary Guidelines for Americans* (4th edition) for the first time. Although a sip of wine for health is suggested in the Bible (1 Tim. 5:23), no one is encouraging anyone to take up drinking. There is evidence, however, that alcohol, particularly red wine, in moderate quantities may protect the heart. The recommendation for moderate consumption is defined maximally as 12 ounces of beer or 5 ounces of wine or 1.5 ounces of 80-proof distilled spirits per day.

Since women tend to be more secretive about their drinking than men, there are many women who successfully hide serious problems with alcohol. Because of a woman's generally smaller size and female hormones, alcohol is a more potent drink for her than it is for a man. In addition to social ramifications, osteoporosis risk factors are escalated because of alcohol's interference with calcium absorption.

Laxatives

A discussion of laxative use may seem an odd topic to include in a book on menopause, but overuse of medication to regulate the bowel often begins at midlife and makes a tremendous difference by old age. Long-term use of laxatives aggravates chronic constipation. Take Bella, for example. Her lifetime use of laxatives has markedly reduced her bowel's ability to function normally. Her family has made six trips to the emergency room because of impacted bowels and the bravest among the daughters has found herself repeatedly helping her mother pick hardened stools from her body. This is not how any of us wish to end our days and yet constant and lengthy use of laxatives ensures we will share Bella's fate.

While a problem with constipation seems a somewhat minor discomfort, it can be life threatening. When stool stays too long in the body, the bowel stretches and toxic buildup causes fainting, dizziness, nausea, and a rapid heart rate, known as a vagovagal response, which can be serious.

For the curious . . . The single most important thing a woman can do to improve her health is quit smoking. Smoking is directly responsible for 21 percent of all deaths from cardiovascular disease in women and 50 percent of all acute coronary events in women younger than fifty-five.

How should you manage constipation?

1. Drink plenty of water.
2. Eat plenty of high-fiber fruits and foods.
3. Set a regular time to go to the bathroom.
4. Try stool softeners (Senakot, Colace) or bulk softeners (Citracel, Metamucil).
5. Occasionally use a suppository or Fleet's enema.
6. For an acute attack, use a laxative temporarily ("Smooth Move" Senna Tea).

Smoking

Unlike the modest exceptions with caffeine and alcohol, there is no tolerable dose of a cigarette, especially if your goal is optimal health. New nonsmoking programs, many covered by insurance, are available. If you have tried to quit before and started smoking again, don't give up; research shows most smokers make several attempts to stop before they succeed. Because of their hormones, women have a more difficult time quitting than men. Additionally, a higher incidence of depression and concern over weight gain complicates the picture.

Nicotine withdrawal is worse toward the end of a cycle; therefore, time your efforts to quit early in your cycle. Since smokers who are most dependent on nicotine often have higher rates of depression, attending to any depressive tendencies will increase the chance of success. Expect an average weight gain of about eight pounds. About 15 percent of women who quit find themselves adding twenty-five pounds or more. It is speculated that nicotine has antidepressant effects triggered by the release of serotonin, norepinephrine, and dopamine, which are also appetite suppressors.

Smoking has a detrimental effect on bone density because it increases the metabolism and breakdown of estrogen in the liver. Women who are heavy smokers are at greater risk than their male

For the curious . . .
Smoking kills more Americans each year than alcohol, cocaine, heroin, homicide, suicide, car accidents, fires, and AIDS combined. Secondhand smoke causes an estimated fifty-three thousand deaths annually in the United States.

More than three billion dollars is spent annually on advertising cigarettes, even with no money allotted to radio or television advertising.

counterparts because of this estrogen factor. For the same reason, smokers lose the protection of estrogen and have reduced production of high-density lipids (HDL). The younger the smoker, the more the risk incurred. A 1996 study presented at the American Association for Cancer Research annual meeting in Washington, by Bogdan Prokopczyk, Ph.D., found tobacco-specific carcinogens in cervical tissue of the mother and in the blood of newborns whose mothers were simply around heavy smokers. This is no surprise since the American Cancer Society has reported that non-smokers who work for eight hours next to someone who smokes experience the same negative effects as smoking three cigarettes and they actually inhale higher levels of tar, nicotine, and carbon monoxide than is inhaled by the smoker. Workers exposed on the job are 34 percent more likely to get lung cancer. Besides, smoking causes your face to become leathery and wrinkled, your breath to be bad, and your teeth to be stained.

For the curious . . . Only about half of current smokers recall being asked about their smoking or being advised to quit by their doctors, according to the agency for Health Care Policy and Research.

Pearls of wisdom for eating . . .

1. Diets don't work.
2. Always eat breakfast.
3. Eat a great variety of goods, especially vegetables and fruits, and don't forget protein.
4. Don't eliminate all fat from your diet—eat good-guy fats.
5. Take a daily multivitamin supplement.
6. Take a calcium supplement.
7. Take extra vitamin E.

14

Wellness Moving

Diane stormed into her house, threw her coat on the chair, and ignored her cat. She had just returned from Dr. Mayo's office and she didn't like what she had heard. Her cardiovascular system was in terrible shape. In fact Diane's health had been deteriorating over the last few years. At fifty-five, she was enjoying not having to work, carpool, or make big meals for a houseful of kids. She was very busy with her painting and loved making dresses and dolls for her granddaughters. Physically, however, she had simply "mushed out," as she liked to say.

It hadn't been easy hearing all the things she needed to change if she were to remain active. It took a week before she could let go of her anger at the messenger of her fate. Finally, however, she was able to sit down and talk calmly about what she needed to do. "Dr. Mayo, I'm only up to one thing at a time," she began. "The only thing I know for sure is that I don't want to take hormones. I acknowledge that my fears may be irrational and that estrogen is protective for whatever is wrong with me but I won't take it."

Dr. Mayo spent considerable time with Diane making sure she understood the consequences of her decision not to use HRT and explaining the importance of other health practices that would preserve her health. Diane was adamant that she could only handle one change at a time.

"If that's the case," Dr. Mayo counseled, "make that one thing a good exercise program and give it priority." Diane agreed she could do that—and she did. In fact even he was surprised when she returned six months later. Her laboratory tests and self-report gave her a new lease on life.

Fortunately Diane didn't sign up for the first aerobic program that came to her attention. Dr. Mayo had recommended a personal trainer who knew physiology and had experience helping people with various health problems. Through her stretching and basic conditioning program, she had been able to reenter the world of exercise without doing herself harm or dealing with excessive aches and pains.

She was surprised how quickly her strength increased and how much better she felt, but the real payoff had been her improved cardiovascular health. Even though she had sworn, "only one change at a time," Diane found her increased stamina and health provided motivation to change other habits. She was eating more fruits and vegetables and avoiding saturated fats. Indeed, regular directed exercise had been a miracle drug for Diane.

ADDING THE "NATURAL HIGH" TO YOUR LIFE

Exercise doesn't have to cost money or be unpleasant but it requires time, effort, and discipline. The payoff affects all areas

For the curious . . .
"Exercise increases the brain's alpha waves. Decreased muscle tension, including the heart muscle, is the result of its ability to reduce circulating catecholamines. [Exercise] induces fat breakdown increasing tryptophan and brain serotonin, norepinephrine, and the stabilization or 'up-regulation' of the hypothalamic-pituitary-adrenal axis. These endorphins, or brain morphines, make us feel good, reduce muscle tension, and decrease anxiety. Epinephrine and norepinephrine improve neurotransmission of nerve messages. As a result, every part of the body is enhanced."[1]

of your health. Most important for menopausal women is its protection against bone loss, its positive changes in the metabolism of lipoproteins, the reduction of hypertension, the decrease in vasomotor symptoms such as hot flashes, and, of course, its beneficial impact on mental health.[2]

Like Diane, if you'll exercise, your chance of having a heart attack will be reduced. In fact women with the lowest risk factors are those who have exercised for more than ten years. Such women are not necessarily marathon runners. They have walked regularly, gardened, and ridden their bikes. Physically active women are less likely to suffer from colon cancer, endometrial cancer, and breast cancer, especially, during the pre- and peri-menopause.[3] However, even postmenopausal women can reduce their risk of premature death by 30 percent by exercising regularly.[4] A large, fourteen-year study of Norwegian women reported that women who exercised regularly for three to five years had the lowest rate of breast cancer even when adjusted for age, body mass, diet, and number of children.[5] Exercise modifies insulin sensitivity and has been shown to reduce the need for insulin. Moderate exercise even enhances the immune system.

For the curious . . . One single episode of rigorous exercise has been shown to reduce anxiety and the body's accompanying fight-or-flight response for two to four hours.

But as important as the physical impact of exercise is, the psychological benefits can be even more striking and immediate.

Regular weekly programs that included physical activity for at least twenty minutes demonstrated that even such minor intervention results in a measurable relaxing effect after ten weeks.[6] Aerobic training three times a week for at least six weeks can be an efficient treatment for mild to moderate depression. In healthy people exercise maintains mental health. People who exercise report a variety of psychosocial benefits such as increased ability to master skills, distraction from daily stressors, decreased muscle tension, improved body image, feelings of competence, and even better interaction with others.

Astronauts lose bone and muscle on confined and lengthy space flights; tennis stars generally have one arm larger than the other. The message is clear: If you don't exercise your muscles, they will weaken and atrophy. On the other hand, excessive exercise—characteristic of anorexics, professional athletes, and dancers—can alter ovarian function and reduce or stop periods, resulting in increased bone loss.

I DON'T HAVE THE ENERGY TO EXERCISE

Cycles of alertness and sleepiness, hunger and cell division, body temperature and heart rate occurring over a twenty-four-to-twenty-five-hour period are known as circadian rhythms. Most people are not exclusively morning or night people. Most of us are somewhere in between, although the majority find working on projects that require thinking, planning, organizing, creating, and making decisions is best done in the morning. Repetitive physical tasks are more efficiently handled in the afternoon or early evening. Athletes are often at their peak between 4 and 6 P.M. According to exercise physiologists, the best training time is around 5 to 7 P.M. Hooking into your natural rhythm results in fewer injuries.

Our bodies have been made to function in a neat and orderly way, but our highly stressed lifestyles alter normal rhythms by changing hormones and actions of neurotransmitters. So when should you work out? Experience tells us that people who work out in the morning tend to be more consistent. But do what fits your lifestyle. Keep your gym bag in your car for that unexpected opportunity to go to the gym or to take a hike.

I DON'T HAVE TIME TO EXERCISE

If you think you don't have time to exercise, do not despair. The American College of Sports Medicine has come to your rescue. They say you don't have to put in three grueling hours daily at the gym to benefit from exercise. An accumulation of at least thirty minutes of moderately vigorous activity on all or most days is adequate as long as you aren't planning to enter any "Iron

Jane" contests. If you don't have thirty minutes, the experts tell us, three ten-minute sessions throughout the day will do. Remember many everyday tasks can be considered exercise; a gym outfit and cross-trainer shoes are not necessary to make it officially count.

"Moderately vigorous" means that while exercising you can still give directions to your secretary, remind your kids to put gas in the car, and call your husband. You can talk but you'll feel the effect on your heart rate and respiratory rate and you'll perspire slightly. That would place the average fifty-year-old at 60–70 percent of maximal oxygen uptake, or a heart rate of 100 to 120 beats per minute.

It doesn't matter if you do aerobics or work out on exercise machines. The important thing is that you do something. If you enjoy it, you are more likely to continue it. Ideally, include both aerobic exercises (that make your heart and lungs work) and anaerobic exercises (that build strength and flexibility). Here are five ways to get more exercise.

1. *Walk*. Park your car and walk a block to your destination. Consistency is important, so incorporate extra walks into your normal routine to get in thirty minutes a day. Bond with your dog—borrow one if you don't have one—and learn to feel guilty when you miss a mutual romp. Wear good shoes, leave those extra weights behind (they hurt your joints), and with each step, place your heel down first.

Think about it . . . Good news: The more out of shape you are, the greater the benefit you will derive from walking.

2. *Take a stretch class*. Beginning ballet, yoga (the exercise version), t'ai chi, stretch classes, or stretching on your own enable you to move your joints through their full range of motion and are excellent for relaxation and reducing stress.

Stretching changes the way muscles respond to nerve impulses and alters muscles and surrounding connective tissue in a way that increases elasticity. Despite their gentle facade, stretch exercises build strength and improve balance and stability, while pre-

200

venting you from creaking and aching when you get out of bed in the morning. Studies show that t'ai chi worked better than high-tech, computerized exercise programs in helping improve balance and reduce falls in older exercisers.[7]

The nicest thing about stretching, however, is that you can do it anytime in anything you happen to be wearing—no lycra required.

- Don't think of stretching as a warm-up to exercise; it is important in its own right.
- Don't stretch to the point of pain, just to tightness.
- Don't bounce.

3. *Fool yourself into thinking you are not exercising.* Take a dance class: jazz, square dancing, western dance, any kind you enjoy. Take up a sport like golf, tennis, racquetball, or swimming.

4. *Join a gym.* Begin your workout with twenty minutes on the treadmill followed by a series of machines designed for strengthening. Let a trainer determine a routine that fits your goals. Always start slowly; it will save time in the long run—pain is not gain.

5. *Convince a friend to join you.* Depending on how you look at it, misery loves company or in the words of the famous philosopher Winnie the Pooh, "It's much friendlier with two."

I'M IN GOOD SHAPE (EXCEPT FOR MY HIPS)

Despite what the infomercials and the endless variety of gimmicks promise, you can't reduce a single spot—you must reduce everywhere. However, strengthening muscles may pull fat in and make you look better. Since all your muscles and joints are connected, you can't impact one area without affecting other parts. Too great a focus on developing "abs of steel," for example, may cause you to neglect and undermine lower-back strength.

As for other exercise myths? You can't sweat fat off. When you sweat, you simply lose water. Muscle does not become fat and fat won't become muscle. When you stopped walking to

201

work, taking the stairs, or chasing a baby, your muscles didn't turn to fat. They simply shrank.

I DON'T WANT TO BE A HARD BODY

Don't fret that lifting weights and using exercise machines will turn you into something only a mother could love. Without steroids, it doesn't happen. You can refine and tone your shape and increase your strength. The good news is that the lean muscle you add speeds up your metabolism and continues to burn calories by just existing. Build strength by using a low-weight, high-repetition program and do each move slowly and deliberately. Remember, however, that if you are working so hard you can't talk, your muscles are unable to get the oxygen they need for proper function and repair.

Experts recommend strength training only three times a week with time between for your muscles, tendons, and connective tissue to repair and rebuild, remove waste products, and replace energy stores. Ironically, strength exercises done too frequently can lead to a loss of strength rather than a gain.

For the curious . . . Adding three pounds of muscle increases the resting metabolic rate by up to 7 percent and daily calorie requirements by up to 15 percent. In other words, the more muscle you have the more calories you burn.

WHAT ABOUT YOGA?

It isn't necessary to become a Hindu or to embrace Eastern mysticism to do yoga exercises. Yoga is always great for stretching. It has been shown to help balance the endocrine system, which in turn impacts hormonal and glandular systems in such a way that a person's health can improve. Retention of water and salt is reduced due to the exercise's ability to modify hormone levels. Western scientific studies support the fact that women who exercise have fewer hot flashes.

In yoga, postures such as the "shoulder stand" appear to relieve problems with temperature regulation. "Inversions," as they are called, alter the flow of blood to the organs in a measurable way. Changing positions tricks the body into believing blood pressure has gone up and it reacts by relaxing blood vessels and consequently lowering blood pressure.

Pearls of wisdom for exercise . . .

1. Exercise improves body and mind.
2. Anything you do to move around is good.
3. Exercise can be effective even if it is done three times a day in ten-minute segments.

15

Wellness Thinking

Dr. Mayo has Gilbert's disease, a congenital form of jaundice, that affects his life in only one way—when he is under unrelenting stress (like delivering ten babies in a row), he turns green, or more accurately, a kind of sickly green-toned pallor. The joke in our family is that, like the Muppet Kermit the Frog, "It isn't easy being green." Chances are you don't turn green when you are stressed. Nevertheless, your body *is* reacting to the increased pressure you are feeling.

You don't have to look far to find signs of stress. It's the increased achiness you feel when you get up in the morning, the cold you can't shake, those feelings of tiredness and depression, rumblings along the intestinal tract, coming down with one "bug" after another, blood clots, chest pain—maybe even a heart attack. Stress lives up to its Latin derivation that means "to be drawn tight."

For sure, stress is not just in your mind. When you are stressed, you release chemicals that contribute to the above conditions and more. Nowhere is this more evident than in your cardiovascular health. It is estimated that more than one-third of all heart disease cannot be explained entirely by preexisting physical factors. For those who suffer from cardiovascular disease, the *Journal of the American Medical Association,* in 1996, reported that mental screening was a better predictor of who was most likely to have a heart attack (and possibly die) than the results of running a treadmill. Those with stress-induced ischemia, or decreased blood flow, were three times more vulnerable.[1]

Surveys reveal that the vast majority of doctor visits are due to stress-related disorders. They are among the top ten reasons

Americans miss work, according to the Occupational Safety and Health Administration. For many American women, not having enough time to meet the demands placed on us by ourselves and others produces the greatest stress. It is this tendency toward what has been referred to as codependency, "overcaring," or an overindulged need to nurture that is so critical to a midlife woman. In fact any strong feeling that life is out of control takes its toll.

IF YOU ARE GOING TO SUFFER ANYWAY, WHY PRACTICE?

The degree to which stress affects your health is not determined by how much stress you have, but whether or not you feel powerful enough to deal with it.[2] In other words, the way you look at what is happening to you makes a tremendous difference in maintaining good health.

Take Maureen, for example. Her mother's deteriorating health has caused her to miss work several times. She is in the midst of leading her company through a major merger. Everyone at work is worried about what the coming changes will mean for them. Maureen's brother objects whenever she attempts to make new, more permanent arrangements for their mother, but he is unwilling to do his share. Her mother is becoming increasingly confused and fearful she will be "put away."

Maureen has been unable to sleep, has become extremely sensitive to food, and has gained ten pounds in three months. She is even tempted to smoke again, despite her pride in having previously quit a lifelong habit.

Outwardly, Maureen's face is taut and she is all business. Fellow workers admire what they view as her strength and stability. Inwardly, her inability to communicate about her situation or to see a resolution is stimulating her brain's autonomic nervous system. This prompts the adrenals to pump extra stress hormones, primarily adrenaline and cortisol, into her bloodstream.

Her hormones do what they were intended to do—her blood pressure increases and her heart races to prepare her to face the

205

challenge her body is signaling. But her crisis does not occur and then subside. Instead, her body remains on full alert. The sustained strain of the blood forcing its way through the vessels damages the arterial walls, making them susceptible to plaque deposits and blood clots.

An abundance of cortisol slows Maureen's metabolism, increasing her serum levels of cholesterol and fat, which elevate her cardiovascular risk. Her hormonal system remains unbalanced, resulting in weight gain and decreased immunity. The day Maureen blew up at her brother—just a five-minute, over-the-edge confrontation—her immune system was almost wiped out for the next five hours.

LIFE IS HARD—GET OVER IT

Indeed, life is difficult. If Maureen expects it to be different, her expectations will add to her stress. So the secret remains: If you can't change it, learn to live with it. Life's crises are going to occur. The only thing you have power over is facing them in a way that does not allow them to become a hazard to your health.

Research confirms that it is not the big things that do us in. Rather we are most harmed by our mood fluctuations resulting from the small, daily negatives we must deal with. It is these small fluctuations that are most highly correlated with disease.[3] Stress reduction techniques, like taking deep breaths and counting to ten, are rarely successful, especially in the throes of a crisis.

There is a Hebrew Scripture that states, "A cheerful heart is good medicine, but a crushed spirit dries up the bones" (Prov. 17:22). "A cheerful heart" does not mean having an unrealistic "Pollyanna" view of life. According to researchers at the Institute of HeartMath (a nonprofit think tank dedicated to uncovering and teaching links between heart function and mental and emotional balance, personal efficiency, and immune system health), a cheerful heart really is good medicine.

While our entire body generates measurable electrical impulses, HeartMath researchers focused on the electricity that flows from the heart to the brain. They confirmed an amazing thing. The bioelectricity of the heart is forty to sixty times

206

stronger than that from the brain. The heart essentially has "a mind of its own," and the electricity it generates not only influences the working of the brain but impacts every cell of the body. Apparently common expressions such as "I'm heartbroken," "That makes my heart ache," "Joy fills my heart," or "I know in my heart . . ." have real biochemical meaning. By influencing the higher brain centers through the baroreceptor system, the heart exerts power over our perceptions, reaction speeds, and decision-making ability—and thus our ability to come to creative solutions.

When people become upset and angry, the sympathetic nervous system, which orders the body systems to speed up and be alert for an emergency, works in opposition to the parasympathetic system, which attempts to slow things down. When we are feeling stress or negative emotions, these two branches of the autonomic nervous system become desynchronized. The clash of two opposing forces appears to trigger something akin to an electrical short, creating uneven, erratic heart rhythms. Applying a simple technique called "FREEZE FRAME" allows the body to synchronize.

FREEZE FRAME is not a metaphysical state, known only in Tibet, or the end result of months of rigorous training. It doesn't require a special outfit or even a quiet retreat. You don't need to pull your car over to the side of the road, or take more than one or two minutes to do it. Its simplicity, which is even easy for children, belies its effectiveness. It is a means of making the heart merry and thus the body healthy.

The process as described in the book *FREEZE FRAME: Fast Action Stress Relief* is simple. As soon as an individual recognizes that she feels angry or stressed, she is to take a time-out, to "freeze frame" the moment. Attention is shifted directly to the heart, and she is to recall a moment of deep appreciation, caring, or joy—to experience a feeling of love, if you will. Once a FREEZE FRAME has allowed the focus to shift, the woman can ask herself for a better way to handle her situation and how she is to follow through. Since higher aspects of the brain have been tapped, solutions are likely to be novel and enterprising. When

207

the technique is used regularly, it tends to revise one's attitude about life.[4]

Hard scientific evidence demonstrating the link between immune factors and learning to activate sustained positive feelings is not new. Measurable proof of the body's ability to modify levels of hormones as a direct result of the way one feels is new. In a controlled study by the Institute of HeartMath, participants were able to double their own levels of the antiaging, "vitality" hormone DHEA, by practicing another similar Heart-Math technique called "Cut Thru" for one month.

Cut Thru is particularly directed at the habit of "overcaring" and the resultant changes in body chemistry due to worry and anxiety. Overcaring is the state in which our original intent to care for someone or something crosses a fine line and we find ourselves feeling victimized and worried. This elevates our cortisol levels. This, in turn, prevents us from thinking clearly and can cause headaches and PMS–like symptoms. People who used Cut Thru had increased DHEA and a 23 percent decrease in the stress hormone cortisol. Until these techniques were used, such dramatic changes in hormone levels had only been observed when

For the curious . . .
When something emotional happens, large amounts of adrenaline and cortisol are released. The immune system shuts down and the nervous system orders the heart to keep pumping. The changed hormonal balance causes fat cells to be released to provide energy. Unneeded for fight or flight and unused, the fat cells are changed in the liver to cholesterol, which, in the general circulation, latches onto coronary artery walls, causing plaques and arteriosclerosis.

subjects were treated with additional hormone medication. This is proof that emotions can change hormone levels.

HeartMath's work is so innovative, practical, and well-documented, we recommend you get the details of the program and a list of books, tapes, and even music. You can contact them at 800-372-3100 or write to Planetary Publications, P.O. Box 66, Boulder Creek, CA 95006.[5]

STRESS BUSTERS: TRY RELAXATION TECHNIQUES

1. Take a minivacation: Clear your mind, reduce noise and interruptions, close your eyes, and take deep abdominal breaths, mentally focusing on something or someplace peaceful. Then stretch and exhale deeply.

2. Try autogenics. Autogenics begins much like the minivacation. After you are settled in, begin by giving your body cues so it knows how you want it to feel. For example, mentally focus on your left arm and say to yourself, *My left arm feels warm and heavy,* until it actually begins to feel warmer and heavier. Use this method for every part of the body. If you practice this two times a day for ten minutes, in a few weeks your body will begin to release tension just thinking about the process, or with a very abbreviated version of the technique.

3. Try progressive muscular relaxation. If you are so uptight you have forgotten what being relaxed feels like, this is the technique for you. Begin by getting comfortable, taking a few deep breaths, and then tighten your hand muscles by making a fist. Pay attention to how it feels. Release your hand. Notice that it feels lighter than it did. Systematically, work through your body tensing and releasing the different muscle groups. It will take you about fifteen minutes at first, but with practice, the relaxation response will occur automatically when you consciously think about it.

4. Try simple stretch exercises. You can do them wherever you are, sitting or standing.

5. Allow yourself a few minutes to daydream.

6. Try biofeedback. When all else fails, or you are fascinated by machines, go to an expert in biofeedback. Their machines have sensors that measure your stress response and help you learn what it feels like to relax.

7. Try positive thinking. Watch the messages you say to yourself, like, *My life is out of control. I'll never be able to relax!* Say instead, *I have many things to deal with but I trust I have the wisdom I need to patiently wait as solutions become evident.* Substitute poetic or spiritual affirmations when you catch yourself being negative. The Bible calls this "renewing" your mind (Rom. 12:2).

8. Try sharing with others. Talk to someone or to a group who can be sensitive to your concerns. They can help through empathy, sharing their similar experience, or by pointing out options you may be missing. Stress is worse when we feel we have no choices.

9. Try getting physical. Play like a child.

10. Try eating balanced meals on a schedule.

11. Try penciling in time on your calendar to do nothing at all.

12. Try regular bedtimes.

13. Try aromatherapy. Aromatherapy is gaining increased respect and moving away from being considered a treatment "on the edge." In Europe insurance covers prescriptions for certain aromatic blends.

Fragrances in oils can be used in the bath, with massage, or inhaled. Lavender oil has been recommended as a sleep aid, alone or in combination with other therapies, by the American College of Obstetricians and Gynecologists. Jasmine has been shown in Japanese studies to increase alertness and attention. It is difficult to measure the effectiveness of most aromatherapy since other variables, like relaxing in a tub of warm water and the placebo effect, are also at work. Other herbal aromas helpful in relieving anxiety and fatigue include basil, chamomile, bergamot, and geranium.

14. Try a massage. A massage is more than a back rub. In knowledgeable hands, manipulation of soft tissue increases the circulation of body fluids, gets nutrients to the cells, flushes out

For the curious . . .
When you smell something, odor molecules strike nerves in the nasal passage, which are translated into nerve impulses that stimulate the olfactory bulbs in the brain that are connected directly to the limbic system. The limbic system is associated with memories and emotions. Additionally, certain smells act as fungicides, are anti-inflammatory, and have antiviral and antibiotic qualities.

waste and toxins, and bathes the body in protective lymphatic fluid. Massage is invigorating to both the skin and underlying muscles. Most people find that it energizes and improves their sense of well-being. Especially with the elderly, it improves flexibility and provides healthful touch they may be getting no other way. Since there is a growing knowledge of the benefits of massage, more insurance coverage is available. If you want to know more about therapeutic massage and the health conditions, like diabetes, it benefits, contact the American Massage Therapy Association at 312-761-2682.

The Spiritual Side of Life

It may seem out of place to include a section on spirituality in the middle of a health book but it isn't. In fact author Larry Dossey, M.D., has made a considerable living with a series of books linking prayer with health, including the *New York Times* best-seller *Healing Words*. The Office of Alternative Medicine and other institutions have funded prayer research, and prestigious peer-reviewed medical journals have recently published articles on faith and healing. While no one is suggesting a choice

211

be made between conventional medical treatment and prayer, results of research indicate that both are valuable.[6]

The motivation to turn to an inner life as one ages is not solely the result of a new sense of our mortality. There is more to it than the triggering of some predeath conversion. One would hope that the wisdom acquired from the very act of surviving into our fifties has something to do with it. Whatever the motivation, it is common for spiritual hunger and awareness to increase at midlife.

After years of being distracted by the "tyranny of the urgent," inner nudges toward the spiritual become stinging jabs, and there is little choice but to pay attention to the soul. Having spent a lifetime compartmentalizing life, our task shifts, as we age, to rejoining intellect and spirit. The good news is that such a shift is beneficial to both body and soul and therefore essential for optimal wellness.

David Larson, M.D., a psychiatrist and president of the National Institute of Healthcare Research, an organization that studies religion and medicine, has reviewed more than two hundred studies to verify connections between religious faith and health. His results were impressive. More than 75 percent of the studies demonstrated links between religious practices and a variety of health conditions. For example, among ninety-

Think about it . . .
On a scale of 1–5, with one representing being out of balance and five perfect balance, where are you? While we can't escape the obligation and roles we play, midlife is a time to look at our lives and reprioritize. Our goal is to be refreshed not tired. Do you really want to continue at the same pace as before? What will happen to you and your relationships if you don't make some changes?

two thousand people who had attended church one or more times per week, there were 50 percent fewer deaths from coronary heart disease, 56 percent fewer deaths from emphysema, 74 percent fewer deaths from cirrhosis, and 53 percent fewer suicides.[7]

Among elderly patients undergoing elective heart surgery, those who categorized themselves as deeply religious and who derived strength and comfort from their religion were more likely than others to be alive six months after surgery.[8] Patients who attend church frequently or pray regularly have lower rates of heart disease, hypertension, and suicide and live longer than those who do not. Those who engage in regular meditation practices see a lessening in chronic pain, cardiac arrhythmias, insomnia, anxiety, depression, and side effects of cancer.

To ignore our spirituality is to leave untapped a major resource for healing. American psychotherapist Sonya Friedman once proclaimed, "When you get right down to it, maturity is the cure for our fatal flaws." Dr. Friedman didn't know how accurate she was.

How Do We Reintroduce Soul into Our Lives?

Introducing or revitalizing the spiritual side of life does not require a retreat to the nearest monastery, a trek across the mountains, or hours of contemplative time alone. Life as we live it can be adjusted to make time for a richer inner life if we begin to pencil activities into our Day-Timers according to our longings rather than being enslaved by our social calendar or what we feel is expected of us.

Rearranging one's schedule to incorporate the sacred is easier than you may think. Thomas Moore in his book *Care of the Soul*[9] suggests the following:

The Sacred of the Everyday

1. Find a space, thing, or spot that nurtures—a place where you feel at peace, safe, and comforted.

2. Add tradition or rituals from your past—our own traditions and rituals are helpful but are not always as deeply satisfying as joining in with time-tested ones that have been shared by segments of humanity with whom we feel particular kinship.
3. Acknowledge and gain new appreciation for your heritage—feel connected to your roots, country of origin, faith tradition.
4. Listen to your dreams.
5. Don't use TV as the "cocktail of the 90s"—a means to "zone" out and let the world pass you by.
6. Get out and walk.
7. Reconnect with nature—real plants, real flowers, pets: Get outside.

Spirituality and religion are too often untapped resources for emotional and physical healing. At midlife there is both reason and motivation for change. Good emotional health enables a woman to stay strong despite difficult circumstances. How well a woman responds to the setbacks of the menopausal period is the issue, not how well she escapes them.

Stressors of midlife are real and made more intense by the multitude of health and societal changes that accumulate at menopause. Richard Nelson Bolles, American writer and educator, has said, "Your life is like a tapestry, being woven by God and history on an enchanted loom. Every bobble of the shuttle has meaning, every thread is important." The Bible speaks of stress increasing faith and the importance of persevering in becoming a person of depth and character. Faith in a loving God, whose power is greater than our own, allows us to release to God many of the worries, fears, and frustrations we carry around. That release can be life changing. And the choice to grow and learn from difficult circumstances and trying times is always available.

The unhappiness and discomfort some women experience around menopause is a motivating force to make changes and reorder life to include what relieves both physical and emotional symptoms. A sense of well-being comes from feeling there is some control over the circumstances of one's life and in the belief that options are available. Good mental and physical health is a combination of physical, biochemical, emotional, and spiritual factors. Therefore, interventions that are beneficial come from a variety of sources.

Pearls of wisdom for reducing stress . . .

1. Handling stress does not mean getting rid of all that produces stress in your life. It means learning to keep your body calm and your attitude positive while you deal with the realities of life.
2. Menopause is a great motivator for reevaluation and elimination of those things that keep your life joyless and out of balance.

PART FOUR

CONSIDERING
BOTANICALS
AND HORMONES

We are all products of how we have lived our lives. At menopause life patterns that you have developed and seemingly gotten away with for years catch up with you. The damage done is cumulative, and problems begin to manifest themselves as the wear and tear on the body takes its toll. Some argue that the prevailing attitudes about women and aging in our society predispose women to experience menopause negatively. It has been said that if we valued ourselves more, we would appreciate our hot flashes, have plenty of energy, be wearing out the man in our life, and feel and express power in all arenas of life. Others claim that menopausal symptoms are manifestations of women mourning their inability to bear children. Some imply that midlife women look at the media message of youth, vitality, and sex and respond by shutting down sexually, loathing their expanding and wrinkled body, and lamenting their fate.

Sometimes we complicate the obvious. There is little hard evidence that women suffer at midlife because they have developed either a psychosomatic response to society's attitudes or have failed to live up to their own "inner goddess" potential. While the paradigm through which one views life is important, it is not the "smoking gun" of menopause. Women at midlife report that they don't feel well and/or that their body is responding differently than it used to. There are physical explanations for why this is so—and this section addresses what you can do about them.

16

The Lesser-Known Options

BOTANICALS, DHEA, AND ANDROGENS

Our son intuitively knows how to resolve computer problems. When he has unraveled some mystery from cyberspace in record time, he is not always able to tell you the details of how he did it. His officemate, when facing a problem, precisely and methodically notes each step toward resolution. In the end, they both solve the problem. Seeing these two in action reminds me there is more than one way to overcome an obstacle. This is certainly true with menopause—many options exist that can make a difference, whether used alone or in combination with hormones.

Certain botanicals have proven helpful in relieving some menopause symptoms. A caution is in order, however. The use of botanicals must be carefully monitored, just as conventional medications should be. Also the purity and bioavailability are tremendously important. Previous shortcomings of using plants as medicines, tonics, and adaptogens (herbs that normalize function generally, while not causing further body upset) are rapidly being addressed. Appendix C contains a list of questions you should ask about the natural products you select.

Botanicals, like vitamins and minerals, often work best in combination and in balance with one another. Relief is not always immediate. You must be patient as your body heals and rebalances, which may take several weeks. Besides normalizing body function, botanicals cleanse, provide nutrition, raise the level of energy, and stimulate the immune system. But it is possible to feel the immediate effects of some herbs, particularly those best known for muscle relaxation, general calming, and allergy or hot flash relief.

You must always consider that your body may react uniquely to individual herbs. Chamomile, for example, a popular tea recommended as an aid for digestion, can cause an anaphylactic response in some people, and I am one of them. In 10 percent of those taking valerian, there is a stimulant effect instead of a sedative effect.

Avoid completely any product that contains ma huang (Ephedra). Common in "weight-loss" teas, it is also recommended as an antihistamine and decongestant. Acting on the central nervous system, it can cause a dangerous rise in blood pressure and heart rate, a particular concern for anyone suffering from high blood pressure, heart disease, diabetes, or thyroid disease. Large doses can cause anxiety, sleeplessness, tingling sensations, and heart palpitations.

A major appeal of herbs, however, is that in general they are less toxic than conventional pharmaceuticals. There is also a different focus for their use. A prescription medication is frequently designed to alleviate symptoms, whereas natural interventions more often focus on the underlying cause of the disease process.

The job of herbs most often is to enhance function and maximize the body's ability to work as it should, although they can be used in therapeutic ranges as well to alleviate symptoms. Like food, medicinal plants tend to have multiple actions. Their complexity makes isolating the exact constituents of healing difficult, even with the new biochemical analyses, but much headway has been made in the last few years.

Botanical medicine can be put to use in a variety of forms. While some herbs are best used fresh, many are dried and used as infusions (steeped as tea, such as peppermint) or as decoctions (simmered over low heat, such as rose hips). Such preparations are relatively weak in comparison to an extract. Tinctures and fluid extracts are mixed with water, alcohol, or various other solvents. A solid extract is further processed into a soft but solid or powdered form and can be purchased as tablets, lozenges, pastes, and capsules. Creams, suppositories, bath oils and salts, and aromatics are examples of nonoral ways medicinal herbs are used. Use often depends on the paradigm of the herbalist. In Germany and the United States extracts are popular, while decoctions are more common among the Chinese and African traditions. Smokes and compresses are favored among Native Americans.

When choosing a botanical, pay attention to whether the whole plant or only the root, leaf, or flower was used, since different parts of a plant have varying medicinal effects. The strength of botanical medicines is defined in terms of the content or the concentration of specific herbs in them. For example, a typical tincture may be listed as a 1:5 concentration, meaning one part herb in grams and five parts solvent in milliliters. Knowing the company you are dealing with is still your most important safeguard. Despite the ever increasing use of botanicals, a 1992 study reported in the *Food and Drug Law Journal,* which analyzed reports on herb toxicity submitted to the American Association of Poison Control Centers and the Center for Disease Control, did not find enough cases to cause serious concern.[1]

Buy brands that guarantee the highest quality and biochemical activity available. The cost of a botanical product often reflects the human energy and resources that a company invests up front during the selection process of each individual plant and the methods used in extraction of the active ingredients. Whether you take one herb or a combination of herbs, the herb's authenticity, freshness, and quality are important factors to consider. Each company should know where in the world their herbs come from, when they were harvested, and how they were stored. They should include a document that verifies that the herb is indeed what it says on the label (see appendix C). This information concerning a plant's "origin" should be available to the consumer either in the form of the company's promotional literature or by calling the manufacturer.

It is also important to remember that herbs need to be taken at appropriate levels to be of value. A few botanicals have been standardized to a single or combination of active ingredients "clinically shown" to relieve menopausal symptoms. Be certain that a standardized herbal extract is taken in sufficient quantity to deliver the active ingredient consistent with the amount shown to be effective from the research. The standardized extract approach is very similar to a pharmacology model and is very symptom specific. Sometimes the cost of standardized herbal ingredients makes it difficult to combine them with other herbs considered important to ensure the maximum success of the standardized extract. With some exceptions, the traditional approach of using combination botanical formulas is preferred because there is greater focus on an herb's ability to work synergistically with other herbs. There is less emphasis placed on eliminating a specific symptom and more emphasis on the overall wellness and lifestyle habits of an individual.

European herbal practices often focus on standardized extracts of single herbs, like *Cimicifuga racemosa* or ginkgo, whereas Chinese, Indian, Native American, and folk traditions of Europe tend toward combinations of herbs. A balanced formula from a reputable company, a melding of the collective experience of years of herbal practice, and the increasing science of how herbs work can save money, may make the product easier to use, and may make it more beneficial. This was most likely a factor in a recent study by Dr. Bruce Ettinger, 1997 president of the North American Menopause Society, and Dr. Janie Hirata that showed no statistically significant improvement in hot flashes using dong quai. The study will be repeated using a combination of herbs.

Some products, like Fem EstroPlex, mentioned in the chapter on hot flashes, utilize the nutritional support of vitamins and minerals with botanicals to make a supplement uniquely designed to support changes in midlife women. You should be aware of the most frequently used herbs for a menopausal woman's concerns (see pages 69–71). The following list of botanicals is not complete but includes the most common ones that you may use alone or in combination for general health or to relieve specific symptoms. Basically, herbs for women tend to do one of two things:

1. They act as a tonic or adaptogen to improve health by safely and in a most generalized way bettering overall function while

increasing resistance to internal and external stress. Adaptogens are herbs that have a balancing effect on the body, working in whatever direction is needed rather than having one fixed action.

2. They act as a phytoestrogen or phytosterol that exerts a mild estrogenic or progesterone effect. Or, by blocking more potentially carcinogenic estrogen produced by a woman's body or through prescription estrogen, they provide safe symptom relief.

Black cohosh root (Cimicifuga racemosa) contains phytoestrogens and small amounts of salicylic acid (the basis of aspirin) for pain relief. Use 1–2 grams three times a day as tea or 1 teaspoon of fluid extract (1:1) or 250–500 milligrams of solid extract (4:1). Excess can cause nausea and uterine contractions.

Commercially it is marketed for menopausal women as Remifemin. While not a hormone technically, its actions are decidedly estrogen-like in its cardiovascular protection, improved vaginal health, reduction of hot flashes, and relief from depressive and anxious moods. It is somewhat like a "super" phytoestrogen. In a maze of chemical reactions, cimicifuga extract inhibits the production of luteinizing hormone while not affecting follicle-stimulating hormone or prolactin production. In other words, it is not acting exactly like estrogen.

Research studies show that two tablets of Remifemin, two times a day over several weeks result in relief from many of the common symptoms of menopause, even more effectively than control groups using premarin or other medical therapy. Relief of vaginal atrophy and depression were particularly noted.[2] In Germany it is the number one selling herbal product for women. Currently (1997) additional research is underway to see if cimicifuga is protective against osteoporosis.

Chaste tree berry (Vitex agnus-castus) affects pituitary function and thus is believed to affect LH and FSH secretion. Research suggests this herb inhibits production of prolactin, a pituitary hormone. Elevated prolactin has been linked to breast soreness, fibrocystic breast syndrome, and water retention. Use three times a day as tea: Steep 1 teaspoon of ripe berries in 1 cup of boiling water for 10–15 minutes. Or use ¼–½ teaspoon as a tincture.

223

For the curious . . .
1 teaspoon =
    5 milliliters
1 tablespoon =
    15 milliliters = ½ ounce

Dandelion (Taraxacum officinale). Dandelion is very rich in a number of nutrients and has been used in diverse cultures for many years. Its root is believed to aid liver and gall bladder function in a variety of ways. The leaves can be used as a natural diuretic that does not cause potassium depletion. Two to 8 grams of dried root prepared by infusion or decoction may be used as a tonic three times a day, or use 1–2 teaspoons as a fluid extract (1:1) or 1–2 teaspoons of the juice of fresh root or 250–500 milligrams of powdered solid extract (4:1). Use 4–10 grams of dried leaves as a tea three times a day or 1–2 teaspoons as a fluid extract (1:1). Because they require high doses, alcohol-based tinctures are not recommended.

Dong quai root or rhyzome. Chinese angelica (Angelica sinensis or polymorpha). Japanese angelica (Angelica acutiloba). Angelica sinensis has long been regarded by the Chinese as a female remedy and general tonic. Its mild but highly active estrogenic effect and ability to stabilize blood vessels may explain its effectiveness in reducing hot flashes and a number of other menopausal symptoms. Dong quai contains various coumarins, essential oils, and flavonoids that act as a general tonic building up the blood, supporting sleep, and reducing joint pain. It is frequently the main ingredient of teas and capsules formulated for women. Taken in low doses there are few side effects, but some species can result in heightened sensitivity to the sun. Take 1–2 grams three times a day as a tea or powdered root or 1 teaspoon as a tincture (1:5) or ¼ teaspoon as a fluid extract.

Echinacea (purple cornflower) is popular for building immunity. Parts or the whole plant of a variety of species are used. It flushes and stimulates the lymph glands to cleanse toxins from the body. It can shorten the course of a flu or cold. To maintain its effectiveness, do not use echinacea continually. It can cause dermatitis and anaphylaxis in allergic people. During times of illness or poor health use 1–2 grams as a tea or dried root or 325–650 milligrams of freeze-dried plant or ¾–1 teaspoon tincture (1:5).

False unicorn root (Chamaelirium luteum) is considered to be a strengthener for the reproductive system. It contains phytosterols that may be converted into female hormones. Large doses can cause nausea and vomiting. Use three times a day as a decoction: Bring 1–2 teaspoons to boil in a cup of water. Simmer gently for 10–15 minutes. Or use 2–4 milliliters as a tincture.

Garlic bulb (Allium sativum) appears to be protective of the heart—lowering LDL and increasing HDL and reducing blood pressure—and exerting a considerable anti-inflammatory effect. There are suggestions it is anticarcinogenic. Quality is determined by how much of the beneficial component allicin will be made in the digestive tract. Garlic needs an enteric coating so that it is not destroyed by stomach acid and to trap garlic odor deep inside the body. It can upset the stomach and trigger allergies. Include more garlic in your diet. One clove (4 grams) is equal to a daily dose of a commercial product providing 10 milligrams of allicin or a total allicin potential of 4,000 micrograms.

Ginkgo biloba is the oldest living tree species in existence. Its use is recorded in Chinese writings that are more than twenty-eight hundred years old. Ginkgo leaf extract (which is more effective than any one of its active ingredients alone) is the botanical most widely recommended at A Woman's Place. Its effectiveness for short-term memory enhancement helps restore women's confidence that they are not losing their mind. Well researched for its ability to enhance the use of oxygen and glucose, it is a potent antioxidant (it is high in quercetin) for the brain. There are almost no side effects (slight digestive upset and headache, which diminish with use) and no known interactions with other drugs. Its effectiveness increases over time, and benefits are usually noticed in two to four weeks with consistent use. It is also useful for ringing in the ears and circulatory problems.

Choose ginkgo that is standardized for content and activity. Use 40–80 milligram capsules three times a day or 1 ounce per day of standard 1:5 tincture. We recommend that when significant improvement occurs, a woman experiment with dropping back to the lowest dosage that maintains mental clarity.

Ginseng root (Panax ginseng). Korean, Chinese, and Asian ginseng contain thirteen different types of saponins, known for their progesterone-like qualities. In its role as an adaptogen, ginseng supports and enhances the body's ability to function both mentally and physically. It can cause breast tenderness and should be avoided by those with cardiovascular problems. It is recommended for short-term use since too much can cause anxiety. American ginseng is energizing and good for stress. Don't take it before going to bed! With any ginseng there are great problems with quality control. Look for standardized, high-quality extracts, using 4–6 grams daily.

Siberian ginseng root (Eleutherococcus sentiocosus), a cousin to real ginseng, is especially rich in progesterone-like saponins and its adrenal effect helps allay fatigue and daily stress. It appears to modify the alarm phase of the adrenal's fight-or-flight response. Studies have shown that as an adaptogen it helps people endure harsh conditions and improve mental performance. Its ability to increase the sense of well-being despite one's circumstance while regulating blood pressure and improving kidney function make it appear ideal for the midlife woman. It is frequently used for those suffering from chronic fatigue since it deals with the fatigue while improving outlook and immune function, which are believed to be at the heart of such a syndrome. In China and Russia ginseng use has had a long history.

High doses (4.5–6.0 milliliters three times a day) can cause insomnia, irritability, and anxiety. People with rheumatic heart disease should not take Siberian ginseng.

Use this herb three times a day for *up to sixty days, followed by a two-to-three-week break.* Use 2–4 grams of dried root or 10–20 milliliters of tincture (1:5) or 2–4 milliliters of fluid extract (1:1).

Licorice root (Glycyrrhiza glabra). There has been considerable research verifying the effectiveness of licorice root. It contains many flavonoids, which have estrogen-like qualities, and saponin, which stimulates progesterone-like activity. It has anti-inflammatory and antiallergenic properties and is able to counteract the negative effects of cortisol, while promoting the action of its good effects. Overuse of licorice can result in high blood pressure, loss of potassium, and bloating and weight gain due to salt and water retention. It should not be used at all by anyone who is hypertensive or on diuretics (water pills). For most people it is safe to use 1–2 grams of powdered root or 2–4 milliliters of fluid extract (1:1) or 250–500 milligrams of solid extract three times a day. When included in a traditional Chinese herb formula, licorice is considered a "harmonizer" that facilitates the action between herbs and their individual functions. In such combinations it is considered safe for most people.

Motherwort (Leonurus cardiaca). The stalks of this plant are used in making a herbal product that reduces anxiety and is a tonic for the heart. Since reducing stress makes hot flashes less severe and improves cardiovascular health, motherwort is a good herb for the menopausal woman. As a tea it can be drunk three times a day: Use 1–2 teaspoons of dried herb infused for 10–15 minutes. Or use 1–4 milliliters as a tincture.

Saint-John's-wort (Hypericum perforatum) is made from the aerial parts of the plant and has long been known to improve mood, particularly the irritability and anxiety of menopause. It relieves mild to moderate depression but is not a cure for major affective disorders. Because of its few side effects, it outsells Prozac by 7 to 1 in Germany. Take 300 milligrams of St.-John's-wort in a standardized extract (0.3 percent hypericin) three times a day with meals. Foods known to interact with monoamine oxidase (MAO) inhibitors—such as cheeses, beer, wine—and medicines, such as L-dopa—should be avoided.

Valerian root (Valerian officinalis) and lavender flowers (Lavendula officinalis) aid sleep by improving sleep quality and helping reduce insomnia and depression. Valerian has a calming effect, binding to the same brain receptor sites as does Valium. Some people with extreme fatigue may find valerian acts as a stimulant. To avoid liver damage, use only 150–300 milligrams of valerian extract (0.8 percent valeric acid). Combining it with passion flower and hops can enhance its effect on insomnia. One

227

teaspoon of dried lavender can be infused for ten minutes with a cup of boiling water for tea, or place lavender oil on the bedside table or in a bath.

Turmeric rhyzome (Curcumin longa). Turmeric is an anti-inflammatory that does not upset the gastrointestinal tract like aspirin or NSAIDS (such as ibuprofen). It reduces the production of prostaglandin E2 (PGE2), which is a major cause of pain. It has been found to lower cholesterol and improve liver and gastrointestinal function. The best way to take turmeric is to include it in your diet.

Ginger (Zingiber officinale) shares much of the effect of turmeric and is also good for motion sickness. Chinese records dating from the fourth century B.C. tell of its healthful benefits. Ginger powerfully inhibits prostaglandins and influences cholesterol levels. Some people experience relief from migraine headache by taking it. While those in India consume 8–10 grams of ginger daily, 1 gram of dry powdered root is usually recommended. More than 6 grams can cause gastrointestinal upset.

For the curious . . . Since ginkgo improves the vascular system in general, it helps the circulation in your hands and feet and is therefore good for Raynaud's syndrome.

Wild yam rhyzome (Dioscorea villosa) was at one time the major source for production of "natural" progesterone because of its high diosgenin content. To become bioavailable as a "natural" progesterone, it must go through a number of laboratory processes. It is, however, considered a helpful herb for its phytosterol and anti-inflammatory properties. If used as a tincture, take 2–4 milliliters three times a day (see chapter 17).

OTHER SUPPLEMENTATION

Melatonin is secreted naturally by the pineal gland when your eyes notice that it is getting darker. It slows your metabolism, lowers your body temperature, and nudges you into sleep. Melatonin levels drop in the morning and the process reverses. The usual dose is 1 milligram at bedtime, not to exceed 3 milligrams. Not a lot is known about its long-term effects and its effectiveness varies among people. It should not be taken regularly. It can increase depression in those who are prone and shouldn't be taken if you have allergies, immune system problems, or autoimmune illnesses. As yet the optimal dose is not known, although it is often sold in large doses. Be careful of the purity and concentration you are buying. This is not a miracle drug and so far its best use may be in overcoming and avoiding jet lag.

Superfoods are mixtures of vitamins, minerals, and foods (usually expensive) that have been combined into one or several capsules or powders. They often are well promoted through network marketing and touted as "the cure for everything." Purity and bioavailability vary enormously. Blue-green algae, bee pollen, and the many others on the market may indeed help you feel better, since they are very high in bioflavonoids, but be aware they can be allergenic.

Vitamin supplementation has been discussed in chapter 13. Nutritional supplements improve overall wellness, which for the menopausal woman means any intervention—herbal or conventional—or lifestyle change will be more effective. Multivitamins also replace some of the vitamins lost when conventional hormone replacement is used.

DHEA

Supplementation with the hormone DHEA is another possibility for increasing declining hormone levels.[3] As another precursor molecule, DHEA can be converted into the customized steroids the body needs. Since DHEA receptors exist, it also has its own functions within the body. For the midlife woman, the effect is not as direct as replacement of estrogen and progesterone, but the general improvement in health is such that some women continue functioning without additional HRT—especially in combination with other good health practices. For others, it boosts the effectiveness of HRT. Still others find it most effective in combination with natural progesterone for relief of hot flashes and vaginal dryness and for a generally improved sense of well-being.

Just what is DHEA? It is a steroid hormone produced by the adrenal glands that is found most abundantly in the body when we are around twenty to twenty-five years old. Because it declines as we age, DHEA is believed to have properties that keep us young and healthy. It is known, for example, to enhance the immune system and causes laboratory animals to lose weight and acquire a more youthful musculature and attributes. Some researchers have found very low levels of DHEA in people with memory problems, rheumatoid arthritis, osteoporosis, cancer, and heart disease.[4] Several studies exist showing a relationship between DHEA levels and breast cancer.[5]

Like natural progesterone, DHEA requires no patent, which severely limits research, since drug companies are unable to profit from it. Long-term use of DHEA has simply not been studied in humans. DHEA can cause measurable increases in levels of estrogen (estradiol and estrone) and testosterone.[6] This is important since becoming menopausal has been shown to accelerate the decline of DHEA(S).[7] Theoretically it raises progesterone levels because both DHEA and progesterone are from the same precursor, pregnenolone. If enough DHEA is present, pregnenolone is then free to be converted to progesterone.

Although levels of DHEA can be measured in the lab, the results don't reveal who will benefit or at what dose. The range for "normal" varies. But postmenopausal women and women who have had their ovaries surgically removed are often in the very low range.[8]

Currently 5–25 milligrams a day are commonly prescribed for women, 25–50 milligrams for men, in capsule form, although larger doses may be given to people with serious chronic diseases such as cancer, chronic fatigue syndrome, and AIDS. Our experience is that a little can go a long way and that smaller doses are sometimes more effective than larger ones. DHEA can be purchased in the health food store, but to insure freshness and bioavailability have a pharmacist compound it.

At low levels, DHEA appears to be safe. Minor side effects include acne and/or slight increases in hair growth on arms and legs. Too much may damage the liver, so periodic liver checks and retests for DHEA levels are recommended until more is known. If you begin taking DHEA and feel worse, you may need hydrocortisone instead, because your adrenal function is at such a low level, you cannot convert DHEA into hydrocortisone.

There are many characteristics of DHEA that may benefit menopausal women. Its reputation for improving memory, mood, strength, and energy levels is an important consideration for midlife. Its apparent ability to enhance the immune system is protective against midlife diseases at a time when immunity tends to drop. Its unfolding role in maintaining and repairing bone may also prove important. DHEA has been aptly called "the hormone that does it all." For now, however, proceed with caution.

YOU TARZAN, ME JANE

Using herbs to treat symptoms of menopause is not as direct a therapy as adding estrogen or progesterone, but herbs can be effective. Adding DHEA supplies the building blocks for a number of hormones a woman may need. Alternatives to directly adding estrogen and progesterone exist with conventional hormones too. For example, progesterone is not the only choice for balancing estrogen (see chapter 17). Sometimes androgen is just the ticket. However, androgens do suffer from poor press. Women fear that taking a male hormone will turn them into a miniversion of the man in their life. However, not to worry. Both men and women normally produce ample amounts of the opposite-sex steroids.

While a woman's estrogen production decreases by 70–80 percent at menopause, her ovaries continue to produce testosterone at near normal levels, but her overall androgen production is reduced 50 percent. There is a connection between the functioning of the ovary and the functioning of the adrenal gland. A woman needs fully functioning ovaries to have fully functioning adrenals. This connection could very well be linked to their shared embryological beginnings. The loss of androgens at menopause results from a decrease in androgenic precursors—basic chemicals that can be turned into a variety of hormones depending on the needs of the body. DHEA (dehydroepiandrosterone), androstenedione, DHEAS (dehydroepiandrosterone sulphate), and even testosterone are examples of precursors. Replacing them can sometimes be more beneficial than replacing estrogen or progesterone. It has been observed that women who do not suffer from osteoporosis have a higher concentration of adrenal androgens.[9] The enzyme aromatase, which is utilized by androgens, has been found in bone, suggesting it may be used in actual bone formation.[10] What this means is that ovarian estrogens alone are not totally responsible for bone health and another benefit of androgens might be improved bone strength.

Specifically, the androgen testosterone can provide relief of hot flashes and other menopausal symptoms in women who have not had alleviation by estrogen alone.[11] It reduces breast pain, has been helpful for vaginal dryness, increases the libido, and improves the sense of well-being.[12] Testosterone also appears to increase energy and perhaps should be considered by more physicians before assuming the dose of estrogen should be increased. It is important to note that estrogen actions can cause a woman's available testosterone to be bound and thus become less available. While estrogen restores libido for some women, this binding effect should make a physician think twice before increasing a woman's estrogen to restore sexual function. Adding more estrogen may tip a woman's body into testosterone deficiency with the resultant further loss of sexual desire, decreased fantasy, lowered sensitivity to sexual stimulation of the nipple and clitoris, reduced energy, and loss of muscle tone.

Indeed, the best press on testosterone is its ability to restore libido in at least 45 percent of those taking it.[13] Sexual desire, sexual fantasies, and sexual arousal are significantly improved when testosterone is given along with estrogen or added to the estrogen/progesterone mix. This is important because as we previously noted, loss of sexual desire is a major complaint of perimenopausal women—and frequently of their partners. The result of feeling more desire is measurable by improvement in rates of intercourse and orgasm. These can be correlated with an increase in blood testosterone levels.

The most common way women take androgens is in oral form, either alone or with estrogen. Estratest is 1.25 milligrams of estrone and 1.25 milligrams of testosterone. Estratest HS is one-half this strength. It is becoming more common for physicians to combine estrogen, progesterone, and testosterone (Estratest HS with a natural or synthetic progesterone). Testosterone skin patches are also available. High-dose shots are discouraged due to masculinizing side effects and the development of liver tumors. Carefully monitoring the dosage prevents the development of facial hair, acne, and a deepening voice.

Pearls of wisdom about alternative treatments . . .

1. Symptoms of menopause may be appropriately and successfully treated with other than hormone replacement.
2. Symptom relief does not necessarily result in risk reduction.
3. Androgens are not just for men only.

17

Use of Natural and Synthetic Estrogen and Progesterone

By far the most controversial aspect of menopause is the use of hormone replacement. While doctors are accused of seeing menopause as a deficiency disease, many women view it as a natural passage of life that need not be tampered with. The press has made the choice seem complicated and chancy. Radical feminists are convinced hormone replacement is a male conspiracy designed to maintain Barbie clones for men's pleasure. The most cynical among us suggest that doctors are only motivated by money and that the push for hormones is to insure a chronically dependent clientele. The answer to whether or not hormone replacement is a good or bad thing is as diverse as the women reaching menopause.

As a result, while trusting their doctors to give them correct advice on a myriad of medical concerns, the line is drawn at hormone replacement. Doctors are viewed as one-note enthusiasts for hormones and thus not open to alternative ways of approaching a midlife realignment. But doctors' enthusiasm for hormone replacement is not coming out of a vacuum. Their medical journals confirm the efficacy of hormones and, as you would expect, are missing the anecdotal and thus scientifically unprovable options women sometimes experiment with on their own.

THE ABCs OF ERT AND HRT

When estrogen is given, it is referred to as estrogen replacement therapy or ERT. When both estrogen and progesterone are

234

prescribed, it is called hormone replacement therapy or HRT. HRT is also used in a general sense, meaning estrogen, progesterone, or some other form of hormone replacement.

Progestogen is a generic name for a compound having progesterone-like qualities. It is made by your body, produced synthetically in the lab, or found naturally as a by-product in plants such as soy and the Mexican yam. When the name *progestin* is used, it refers to a synthetic progestogen.

Estrogen is an inclusive name for the female sex hormones—estrone (E1), estradiol (E2), and estriol (E3). Besides those produced by the body, there are synthetic versions made in a laboratory. Two synthetic versions exist, one based on chemical engineering and the other manufactured from plants, most frequently soy and the Mexican yam. The most widely used estrogen, Premarin, is extracted from the urine of pregnant mares.

As research on menopause continues, you are likely to hear more about specific types of estrogen. Estriol, estrone, and estradiol are all estrogen but their actions are not always equal. When you were young, the chief estrogen in your body was estradiol. It is the most potent and biologically active of the three. It is also the form considered to be the most carcinogenic.

Menopausal women have a predominance of estrone, the primary type of estrogen made from fat cells. It has been observed that estrone has a higher metabolic clearance rate

For the curious . . . Estradiol is the chief ingredient in birth control pills. Even the lowest dose of birth control pills has four times the estradiol used in ERT.

than estradiol, meaning it is broken down and excreted by the body more quickly. Naturopathic physicians believe estrogen replacement should be made with the estrogen that is most "naturally" present; therefore, if ERT is called for, they would tend to recommend estrone. For these reasons, we refer to estrone as a "user-friendly" choice, particularly when it is manufactured from the Mexican yam or soy. Others argue that no matter what estrogen you put in your body, it will convert to the form the body needs. More research is forthcoming that will clarify precisely how the body uses these three versions of estrogen.

Estriol is not only the weakest version of estrogen, but it is also present in the smallest amount. It received a reputation as anticarcinogenic from a study done in which estriol was given to women with metastasized breast cancer. Thirty-seven percent had their cancer stopped or reversed. It is considered to be a "weak" estrogen because it binds to the estrogen receptor for a shorter time and is not there long enough to exert a complete estrogen effect.

Future estrogens are being called designer or smart estrogens because they will have all the positive estrogen effects and none of the negative ones. Drugs are also on the horizon that are not estrogens at all. They are called SERMs for selective estrogen-receptor modulators and would do only the good work of estrogen. Raloxifene (Estiva) is currently being tested as a long-term substitute for the cardiovascular and osteoporotic effects of estrogen, if not its symptom relief from hot flashes and vaginal dryness. Tamoxifen is currently being used for up to five years as hormone replacement and for its anticarcinogenic protection for those with breast cancer. Researchers believe sophisticated drugs designed to turn on some switches but not others within the estrogen receptors will be commonplace in a few years.

Why Women Don't Want Hormone Replacement

- "I don't need them; this is a normal passage, even if it is a rough one."
- "My concerns are not taken seriously."
- "The medical profession is too anxious to provide a global hormone approach to my unique and individual concerns."
- "I'm afraid of the side effects—particularly cancer."
- "I don't have enough information."

Why Women Choose Hormone Replacement

- Currently, the biggest increase in hormone replacement therapy is among perimenopausal women who are making the choice because of the severity of their symptoms.[1]
- Women who use hormones tend to be the most symptomatic.

- High cardiovascular and/or osteoporosis risks motivate some women.
- Women use hormones to counter the effects of naturally occurring, premature, or surgically induced menopause.

Why Women Stop Taking Hormones

- "I'm afraid of cancer." When estrogen replacement was first prescribed for women, it was not taken with progesterone. Unopposed estrogen can increase the risk of uterine cancer by 60 percent, from the normal baseline chance of 6 percent. Since then, estrogen and cancer were forever linked in the public's mind, even though the addition of progesterone actually lowers the risk of uterine cancer to 4 percent—below that of the woman who takes no hormones. Evidence of a possible link to breast cancer revives old concerns (see chapter 19). But—it bears repeating—the greatest health risk women face is not cancer, but cardiovascular disease. Each year over 450,000 women die of cardiovascular disease, accounting for 50 percent of all deaths: 46,000 women died of breast cancer in 1994.
- "My HMO no longer has the hormone that works best for me on their formulary, and I can't afford to buy it." Just as there is growing knowledge of the unique sensitivities of individual women, the choices are narrowing. The various brands and types of estrogen as well as increased use of natural phytoestrogens and progesterone mean more choices are available but a woman may have to pay for her choice out of pocket or do without.
- "I don't like the breakthrough bleeding and I feel bloated." It takes great patience to wait out the "hormone adjustment stage" some regimes require. Subtle differences in manufacturing can make enormous differences within an individual's body. One pill, dose, or regime is not right for everyone.
- "I don't like having periods." There are many different ways to take hormone replacement therapy—some of them eliminate periods quickly (see page 242).

237

- "I don't care what they say, I've gained weight since I've been on hormones." Most menopausal women gain approximately ten pounds over a period of three years, which is more related to aging, a reduced metabolic rate, and lifestyle factors than to hormones. A direct weight increase that can be attributed to hormones is bloating, caused by retention of salt, which in turn causes water retention but this can be controlled by decreasing salt intake, using diuretics, and experimenting with various brands and delivery systems of estrogen (see page 242).
- "I don't like the PMS side effects." Again, different medications affect people differently. Your willingness to keep a menopausal diary of symptoms and be flexible, while the best regime is uncovered, requires patience. Hormones are not magic pills that eliminate all menopause symptoms. Other health interventions such as exercise, stress reduction, and vitamin E must be adhered to for maximum relief.
- "I stayed on it three weeks and didn't feel anything." Hormones are not like aspirin or any other medication that acts immediately. Although some women notice changes within a couple of weeks, others find it takes one to two months or longer before they are aware of any improvement.

When You Should Take Hormone Replacement

- You should use hormones when your risk factors for heart disease, osteoporosis, and perhaps, colon cancer, Alzheimer's, and diabetes, are high, and hormone therapy would be protective.
- You should use hormones, even without high risk factors, if your symptoms of menopause are severe enough to affect your quality of life, and other more natural interventions have been tried and provided little or no relief.
- Hormone use is called for in some women who are symptomatic after a premenopausal hysterectomy and is highly recommended if the ovaries are removed.
- You should use hormones if you are experiencing premature menopause.

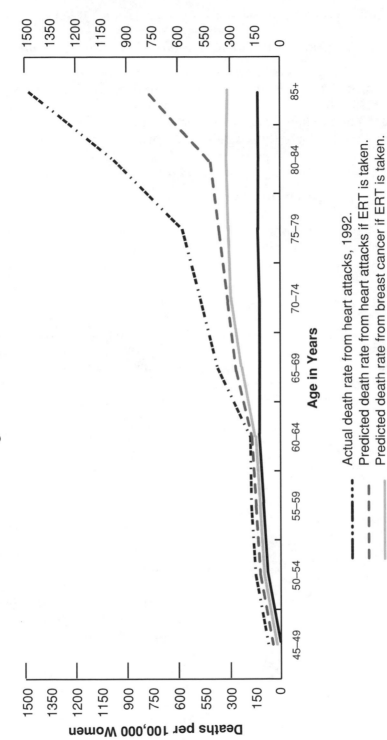

Assessing the Risks and Benefits of ERT

Deaths per 100,000 Women

1500 1350 1200 1150 900 750 600 550 300 150 0

Age in Years

45–49 50–54 55–59 60–64 65–69 70–74 75–79 80–84 85+

Actual death rate from heart attacks, 1992.

Predicted death rate from heart attacks if ERT is taken.

Predicted death rate from breast cancer if ERT is taken.

Actual death rate from breast cancer, 1992.

Adapted from National Center for Health Statistics,
New England Journal of Medicine and the *New York Times*.

When You Should NEVER Use Hormone Replacement

- You have been diagnosed with active liver disease.
- You have a history of hormone-induced thromboembolism.
- You have a history of embolism not caused by trauma.
- You are having undiagnosed vaginal bleeding.
- You have a history of gallbladder disease, especially gallstones.

When Hormone Replacement Is an "Iffy" Choice for You

- You have chronic liver disease.
- You have been diagnosed with a hormonally sensitive cancer.
- You have severe hypertriglyceridemia.
- You have a history of endometrial cancer.
- There is a history of breast cancer in your mother or sisters.

WHAT DOES THE GOVERNMENT SAY?

I'm sure you will be pleased to know that the U.S. Office of Technology Assessment has decided that hormone replacement therapy for everybody costs less than treating just those who develop osteoporosis. The government is indeed all heart. "HRT given to all women at menopause is more cost-effective than screening all menopausal women for low bone density and treating only those at highest risk for osteoporosis."[2]

For the curious . . . Internationally, English and Italian women use fewer hormones. Germany has the highest usage and in the United States, you are less likely to use hormones if you live on the East coast; more likely on the West coast.

HOW SHOULD YOU TAKE HORMONE REPLACEMENT?

If your risk factors, personal philosophy, and financial considerations have led you to hormone replacement therapy, there are still choices to make. You must decide what kind of estrogen and progesterone is best for you and the method of using it that will result in your greatest health benefit.

240

Three basic types of estrogen are available:

1. Premarin, derived from pregnant horse's urine, contains all three estrogens.
2. Pharmaceutically produced estrogen may be synthetic or a derivative of the Mexican yam or soy.
3. "Natural" phytoestrogens derived from the Mexican yam and soy are compounded into creams, gels, lozenges, and capsules by individual pharmacists.

For the curious . . . A woman celebrating her sixty-fifth birthday in 2050 can anticipate 23.1 more years of life to age 88.1 years.

Two basic types of progesterone are available:

1. Synthetic progestins
2. "Natural" progesterone in bioavailable creams and gels or micronized progesterone capsules, lozenges, and oil drops

Hormone replacement gets into your body in the following ways:

- Orally as pills or capsules
- Transdermally as patches
- Sublingually as drops or lozenges
- Intramuscular injection
- Creams and gels as in vaginal and skin creams
- Intrauterine device/vaginal rings
- Pellet implants

Estrogen is rarely given without progesterone to women who have their uterus, except for those who are particularly sensitive to progesterone/progestin or who have other medical or personal reasons for not using both hormones. The risk of using estrogen alone is reduced with low doses and careful monitoring of unscheduled bleeding. Women on their own, however, buy products containing progesterone without prescriptions, usually in a cream or gel form (Progest cream and yam cream). It is a mistake to assume these products will provide protection from uterine cancer, although they can provide symptom relief in some women.

THE "PILL" FOR THE SECOND HALF OF LIFE

The most common way of taking hormone replacement is through pills. In the past, estrogen and progestin were most frequently prescribed in a fashion that mimicked a normal menstrual cycle. Today it is not unusual to take HRT continuously, but there are many variations. In 1996 the first tablet was released that contained both estrogen and progestin: Prempro for continuous use and Premphase for sequential therapy. Oral HRT must first go through the digestive tract and liver before entering the bloodstream.

Typical Hormone Schedules for Pill Takers

Regimen	Estrogen	Progestogen
cyclic sequential	days 1–25 of the month	days 13–25 of the month
continuous sequential	every day	days 1–14 of the month
continuous combined	every day	every day
cyclic combined	days 1–25 of the month	days 1–25 of the month

OTHER WAYS TO TAKE HORMONE REPLACEMENT THERAPY

There are several other methods for taking HRT:

- *Estrogen injections.* For some women, the effects of estrogen are only realized through intramuscular injections. Because of their oil base, shots of estrogen are slowly absorbed and last an extended time, usually one to two weeks. Self-injection can be taught.
- *Transdermal patches.* The patch is a 1–2-inch self-adhesive material through which small amounts of hormone are continually released. Hormones enter the bloodstream through tiny blood vessels near the skin's surface and begin circulating throughout the body without first passing

242

through the liver. There are many varieties on the market. The patch is generally replaced once or twice a week depending on the brand and its placement must be alternated between the buttocks and abdomen to avoid saturation of the area and to prevent a red circular mark caused by dilated small capillaries.

- *Lozenges, drops, gels, and creams.* Like the patch, these delivery systems transport the hormone immediately into the bloodstream. Some women complain that the lozenges placed under the tongue leave a fatty film on the inside of their mouth. Creams have the disadvantage of delivering the least accurate dosage. Gels are proving to be a better delivery system that is more accurate than creams and without the problem of skin irritation associated with the patch.
- *Pellet implants.* Pellet implants are inserted in the subcutaneous tissue. The good news is their steady release and long-term availability, up to six months. The bad news is a small scar because a surgical procedure is necessary to insert the pellet.

So What Is the B-E-S-T for H-R-T?

It is impossible to know what is best for every woman who, along with her physician, determines she would benefit from hormone replacement. Unfortunately the only true test is trial and error. Our experience has been that even subtle changes in pill coating can alter the rate of delivery and affect a woman's acceptance and benefits. Both experience and research reveal that if a woman does not feel measurably better on HRT, she will not stick with it, despite promises of long-term benefit. Research also indicates that once a regimen is decided on, women continually reevaluate and rethink the wisdom and effectiveness of their decision.

Premarin is the most widely prescribed and best-researched estrogen. For some, this is a concern. Its benefits result from the fact that it is "conjugated," meaning it contains estrone, estradiol, and estriol, which are the three types of estrogen found in every woman's body. New studies on premarin suggest that equilin, which is also found in this "naturally" occurring hormone,

243

increases blood flow to the brain more effectively than synthetic versions.[3]

SOME OBSERVATIONS

After four to six months with continuous HRT combined therapy, 60 percent of women will not bleed. Those who continue to bleed will need to consider a sequential regime.

For those on a cyclic combined regimen, low doses of estrogen and progesterone are given from day 1–25. Spotting will usually occur the first month but for most women it stops by four months, after which breakthrough bleeding may occur on the twenty-sixth or twenty-seventh day, allowing only two days of spotting. Discontinuing the progesterone allows for shedding any endometrium buildup with few side effects.

For women who have been without a period for more than one year, well-known obstetrician-gynecologist, researcher, and author, from the New York School of Medicine, Dr. Lila Nachtigall recommends continuous combined treatment with estrogen and progesterone or with an estrogen/androgen and progesterone.

Headaches and other side effects of progesterone are eliminated or reduced by as much as 50 percent when low doses of diuretics (spironolactone, hydrochlorothiazide, or dandelion root) are given seven to ten days before menses along with progesterone.

A cyclic sequential combined hormone schedule (estrogen taken every day, progesterone added the first through the fourteenth day of the month) has been noted as having the fewest side effects; however, most women continue to have periods with this regime. Fluid retention and breast pain may be relieved with a cyclic schedule. At M. D. Anderson Cancer Center this is considered the most effective hormone replacement.[4]

Some synthetic progestins have less withdrawal bleeding and fewer side effects than others, depending on the individual. Fewer side effects (PMS–like symptoms) are found in the 25 percent of women who are particularly sensitive to synthetic progestins when they take micronized "natural" progesterone.

The long-term effects of continuous combined therapy are not yet known. There is some increase in endometrial cancer noted after two to four years of low dosage, continuous combined use.

The protective effects of HRT are dose and duration dependent. When you quit using it, the protective effects will not continue.

HRT replacement needs and levels vary as you encounter the everyday vicissitudes of life. Plan on rechecking your regime and delivery system annually.

HRT is not a magic pill that effectively and completely eliminates menopausal symptoms. It is a tool that must be used along with other healthy practices to create optimal health.

Is discontinuing hormones a cold-turkey nightmare? If you are still having periods or using a cyclic pattern for taking your hormones, in most cases there is no problem discontinuing them after completing a cycle. If you are on continuous therapy, you can stop anytime. It is also appropriate to taper off by extending the days between pills. Symptoms that have been alleviated with hormone therapy will return.

GOOD NEWS ABOUT HRT

Women on HRT live longer. Whether this is due entirely to the beneficial effect of hormones protecting against heart disease and osteoporosis or the fact that such women may have different health habits from those who don't take hormones is difficult to discern. Living longer means getting old enough for cancer and Alzheimer's disease, and for rates of other diseases to naturally increase.

It has been estimated that between 211 and 328 more women per one hundred thousand, aged sixty-five to seventy-four years, could be alive if they had used HRT. This would be the result of fewer hip fractures and less cerebrovascular disease, coronary artery disease, and cancer.[5] If women aged fifty took estrogen for twenty-five years to age seventy-five, 574 deaths would be prevented out of every ten thousand women, and 3,951 quality-adjusted life years could be lived, compared to women who do not take estrogen.[6]

Despite these statistics, at this point in time there is no finite way to define and determine who will positively benefit from

HRT. Even the new, more sophisticated measurements of female hormones do not automatically translate into a checklist of when and what hormones are necessary. The decision is not the physician's alone, but one made in partnership with the woman and requires considerable subjective input. Quality of life issues, personal philosophy, and personality must be combined with laboratory test results and family history to determine whether hormone replacement is the best choice, given current available information, for any individual.

DETAILS ABOUT ESTROGEN

The truth is, in spite of the bad publicity and the problem of finding the right dosage and delivery system with the least side effects, there are good things that can be said about estrogen replacement from a multitude of scientific studies. This is what your physician reads in his or her journals.

For the curious . . . One study found that 20–30 percent of women given prescriptions for HRT never fill them, and 20 percent stop taking HRT within nine months.

Most studies conclude that estrogen has beneficial effects on a woman's cardiovascular system[7](see chapter 12). Minimally, research has shown that estrogen does not increase blood pressure or the risk of stroke and provides a major protective effect against coronary artery atherosclerosis. For women in their fifties, sixties, and seventies a strong relationship exists between high cholesterol, LDL, and coronary disease. The ongoing, most comprehensive study, the PEPI Trial (Postmenopausal Estrogen and Progesterone Intervention), has concluded that estrogen, with or without progesterone, lowers LDL and raises HDL.[8] The greatest increase in "good" cholesterol, HDL, and lowering of "bad," LDL, was produced by estrogen and cyclic micronized progesterone— natural progesterone. It should be noted, however, all ERT and HRT combinations minimally lowered LDL and made the other cardiovascular improvements.

All in all, studies indicate estrogen reduces the incidence of heart disease by 50 percent. The Framingham Study is one of few studies showing a negative effect of ERT on cardiovascular health but the researchers used higher doses of estrogen than was generally used in other studies.

There are other ways that estrogen is beneficial:

- Estrogen protects against osteoporosis. The Framingham Study showed a 35 percent reduction in hip fracture risk among ERT users.
- Estrogen helps keep the urinary system in good working order.
- Estrogen protects against colon cancer (see chapter 18).
- Estrogen maintains higher levels of collagen for healthier skin and bones.
- Estrogen keeps the vulvar and vaginal region plump, moist, and resistant to infection.
- Estrogen can positively affect mood and a sense of well-being.
- Estrogen aids sleep.
- Estrogen can increase sexual desire.
- Estrogen can help with endogenous depression.
- Estrogen can improve memory.
- Estrogen protects against the onset of Alzheimer's disease and improves functioning for those who already have the disease (see chapter 18).
- Estrogen appears to aid in glycemic control.[9]
- Estrogen reduces joint and muscle aches.
- Estrogen appears to be protective against diabetes (see chapter 18).
- Some studies show that estrogen helps prevent the degeneration of cells in the hippocampal area of the brain that is used for balance and coordination.[10]
- A combination of estrogen and progesterone may reduce the risk of some types of breast cancer and recurrence (see chapter 19).
- Estrogen reduces hot flashes.
- Estrogen aids in gum and teeth health.
- Estrogen helps to reduce "dry eye" and cataract formation.

For the curious . . .

Estrogen's positive cardiovascular effect is due in part to:

- Its ability to influence how cholesterol is metabolized. It destroys LDL and produces HDL.[11]
- Improvement in the functioning of cells that line the
  cavity of the heart and blood vessels.[12] Production of
  a relaxing factor that enables the arterial walls to
  remain flexible.
- Estrogen receptors in the smooth muscle cells, which
  determine the flow and stability of blood through
  the system.[13]
- Its antioxidant effect on LDL.[14]
- Its ability to reduce the destruction of other antioxidants known to be good for the heart such as vitamin C, E, and beta-carotene.
- Its ability to inactivate nitric oxide, which is known to
  increase blood flow and pressure and is associated
  with plaque formation on the arterial walls.

WHY ESTROGEN ISN'T A WONDER DRUG

Estrogen produces over four hundred well-documented actions that affect nearly every system. As we have seen, many are beneficial. While this is so, it is clear that any hormone given in an inappropriate dosage can lead to imbalance in the overall body system, causing numerous problems.

When estrogen is given during the perimenopause or menopause, the goal is to find a dose that truly "replaces" what is needed for optimal health—not bathe the system in excess estrogen. In the future, technology will allow even greater precision in monitoring levels and dosage—pinpointing your unique "estrogen zone," for example—and the goal of true "replacement" will be more easily achieved.

The most significant and verified negative associated with estrogen occurs when it is given without the opposing balance of progesterone. Hyperplasia, an overgrowth of the uterine lining, occurs in 7–15 percent of women taking estrogen alone. Hyperplasia is a concern because it can progress to endometrial cancer. Today, unless they have had a hysterectomy, most women take some form of combined therapy. Before the 1980s, however, estrogen was almost always given without progesterone.

The biggest fear of those using estrogen is developing breast cancer. Those whose mother and/or sisters had a diagnosis of breast cancer, particularly under age fifty, need to carefully evaluate the wisdom and risk of HRT in light of their family history, lifestyle, and other risk factors, as outlined in chapter 19. A 1997 article in the *New England Journal of Medicine* examined the relationship between postmenopausal hormones and mortality from information gathered from the Nurses' Health Study. They concluded that ". . . mortality among women who use postmenopausal hormones is lower than among nonusers; however, the survival benefit diminishes with longer duration of use and is lower for women at low risk for coronary disease."[15] The study also indicated that the protective effect of hormones was lost five years after the women quit using them. Death from breast cancer was reduced, but over time there was a slight increase in its occurrence. The observation can be made that if you have a high cardiovascular risk and low breast cancer risk, long-term use of HRT will lengthen and improve the quality of your life. If you have a high breast cancer risk and low risk for osteoporosis and cardiovascular disease, you may have little to gain by taking it. Remember that the incidence and severity of each of the diseases that benefit from the use of HRT can be reduced by lifestyle interventions such as weight control, exercise, and other healthy lifestyle choices.

There may be other side effects of estrogen:

- nausea
- fluid retention
- irregular bleeding
- breast tenderness
- increased chance of gallstones

- may enlarge fibroids although ongoing research is discounting this risk
- bloating
- PMS symptoms
- headaches in susceptible women
- increased abnormal blood clotting and the risk of blood clots

Dr. Leon Speroff, a foremost expert on estrogen replacement and professor of obstetrics and gynecology at Oregon Health Sciences, has reported that increased blood clotting appears to be dose dependent, with lower doses (.625 milligrams) being protective and higher doses (1.25 milligrams) increasing thrombotic problems. This is another indication of the importance of true "replacement-level" hormones.

A "NATURAL" FORM OF ESTROGEN

Phytoestrogens, as they are called, are plant compounds converted to a bioavailable state in the laboratory or by the metabolic processes of the body when plants that contain their precursors are eaten. Lignans and isoflavones are the two main classes that convert to a form that structurally resembles estradiol (E2). Soybeans and flaxseed oil are particularly abundant sources of phytoestrogens, and they are also found in cereal bran, yams, and legumes, among other foods, as well as in some herbs.

Phytoestrogens are not as strong as conventional estrogen but research indicates that when phytoestrogens are used medicinally (and to a lesser extent, consumed), there is relief of menopausal symptoms, reduction in serum luteinizing hormone and FSH, increased serum sex-hormone binding globulin (SHBG), and improvement in vaginal epithelium. In other words, their effects are similar to those of a woman taking conventional hormone replacement. The difference is that they are much weaker and they have the ability to act as an estrogen or in an anti-estrogenic fashion, depending on the hormone balance of the individual. Long-term research in peer-reviewed journals that proves their effectiveness in protecting against heart attack and osteoporosis is limited. However, there is plenty of anecdotal evidence and increasing peer-reviewed evidence that indicates their effectiveness in relieving menopausal symptoms.

When a woman's estrogen levels are high or concentrated, as they are in the breast, phytoestrogens are able to bind to the estrogen receptors, leaving fewer sites (parking spaces) for a woman's own estrogen or other estrogen impostors such as the by-product of the pesticide DDT. The result, at least theoretically, is a reduction in the overall estrogen effect. On the other hand, when estrogen levels are low, phytoestrogens are able to promote estrogen functions. In their ability to balance hormone levels in either direction, phytoestrogens act somewhat like a "female" tonic. Overall, they have about $1/400$th the effect of estrogen made in the body or synthetic estrogen.

To effectively relieve symptoms, not necessarily risk, for patients who prefer natural estrogen, we have our local pharmacist compound a particular combination that is in the best interest of the individual woman. Often it is a tri-estrogen (tri-est) formula, combining 10 milligrams of estrone, 10 milligrams of estradiol, and 80 milligrams of estriol. This combination provides adequate symptom relief for some, with the primary portion being the weakest estrogen, estriol. It is the preferred choice of many women with a family history of breast cancer, since estriol is thought to be anticarcinogenic.

THE DETAILS ABOUT PROGESTERONE

Look on the Internet under "menopause" and you will find several web sites devoted to one-stop shopping for anyone on a menopausal journey. A bit of "surfing" and you are quickly aware the tour guides for your trip have apparently consulted the same travel brochure. Repeatedly the benefits of progesterone, particularly "natural" progesterone, are interspersed with dire warnings of "estrogen dominance." No matter where you are in your journey, your path will be made straight, they declare, simply by purchasing one of the advertised, "superwhammy-guaranteed-to-get-you-there" progesterone products.

251

For the curious . . . Using unopposed progesterone daily increases bone loss; used cyclically (ten days a month), its effect is positive.[16]

Progestogens gained popularity when they were found to decrease the incidence of endometrial hyperplasia (overgrowth of the uterine lining). They work by inhibiting both estrogen receptors and cell division in the lining of the uterus. Progesterone is responsible for endometrial shedding and therefore is the primary cause of bleeding irregularities and the occasional resumption of periods while on HRT. In fact after one month of HRT, withdrawal bleeding occurs in as many as 97 percent of women, until age sixty, when it drops to 60 percent. Fortunately, when compared to periods earlier in life, these continuing menses are, in most cases, light and less painful. While there are numerous estrogens on the market to choose from, there are few choices of progestogens. In Asia, Europe, and Australia, a new progestogen, dydrogesterone (Duphaston), has a molecular structure closer to natural progesterone, is bioavailable when taken orally, and results in greater cardiovascular improvement and less breakthrough bleeding than Provera, the most commonly prescribed progestin in the United States.[17] Crinone, soon to be marketed by Wyeth-Ayerst, is an intravaginal progesterone gel that is well-absorbed and has the benefits of natural progesterone.

There is accumulating indirect evidence as well as some long-term studies that show that the addition of progesterone decreases breast cancer risk.[18] Progesterone has been shown to reduce the severity of hot flashes.[19] Estrogen and progesterone are needed to maintain the proper balance of receptor sites for both hormones. Overall, progesterone does appear to positively balance estrogen. Any modifying effect of progesterone on the full action of estrogen against heart disease appears to be modest. Notably, triglycerides do not rise with estrogen/progesterone use but do with estrogen use only. The protective effect of progesterone for other diseases such as endometrial cancer, breast cancer, and osteoporosis warrants its use. The effect appears to be dependent on the route, type, and amount.

While it is too soon to know for sure, combination therapy may have a synergistic action that restores and promotes new bone formation, especially if taken over long periods of time. Since it slows the amount of calcium loss from bone, progesterone is a partner with estrogen in maintaining strong bones.[20] For sure it can be said that the addition of progestogens in combination with estrogens has not reduced the effectiveness of estrogen alone. Higher bone density outcomes in premenopausal women have resulted from using cyclical regimes and in postmenopausal women using continuous therapy.[21] Preliminary reports from the PEPI Trial (1995) indicate that women on estrogen alone, or estrogen plus sequential progestins or natural progesterone, given twelve days per month (continuous usage wasn't tested), did better than placebo groups. Most studies on progesterone have demonstrated a positive effect on bone building not dissimilar to that of estrogen but not as potent.[22]

These preliminary findings are motivating some doctors, and we agree with them, to suggest that their patients take both progesterone and estrogen, even if they have had a hysterectomy. New combination pills (estrogen plus progestin) have been approved, as have new delivery systems such as an IUD (intrauterine device, Progestosert) for progesterone delivery.

WHY PROGESTERONE ISN'T A MAGIC PILL, EITHER

The use of progesterone is not without problems.

Taking progestogens can be one big PMS trip. There are women (25 percent) who have a very difficult time with PMS–like side effects, such as headache, abdominal cramping, irritability, depression, and lethargy, when taking progestogens. Many of these symptoms are related to fluid retention, secondary to the retention of salt. Studies to discover the lowest

For the curious . . .
Progesterone receptors in osteoblast-like cells promote bone formation and/or increase turnover of bone, particularly cortical bone.[23]

253

dose of progestin (the synthetic version) that is still protective against hyperplasia, have shown that 5–10 milligrams given cyclically for twelve to fourteen days or in a continuous combination with 2.5 milligrams progestin daily is a minimum dose. Some women find greater tolerance by using lower dosages of C-19 progestogens, by adding progesterone-rich low-dose birth control pills (Micronor) with the estrogen for the last twelve to fourteen days of the cycle, or by using vaginal suppositories of micronized progesterone, 25 milligrams twice a day for twelve to fourteen days. Natural micronized progesterone, 300 milligrams for twelve to fourteen days divided into a 100-milligram dose during the day and 200 milligrams at night, works well for many women who simply can't tolerate the synthetic version.

There are other problems that may result from progesterone use:

- High doses cause a sedation effect.
- Withdrawal can cause symptoms, such as headache.
- Glucose tolerance may be affected, making diabetic control more difficult, especially in higher doses. However, cyclic progestin appears to have little or no impact on carbohydrate metabolism.
- Abdominal bloating may occur.
- Breast tenderness, which often goes away after an adjustment period, can be *relieved* or *caused* by progesterone.
- Sometimes there is generalized swelling.

"NATURAL" PROGESTERONE

Fueled by fears of estrogen and influenced by the fact that it is considered "natural" because it is plant-based and can be bought without a prescription, many women have opted for natural progesterone for relief of menopausal symptoms. Progesterone's reputation as protective against breast cancer has simply added to its appeal. Such faith is not entirely misplaced, for micronized progesterone provides some advantages over synthetic progestins, including a vastly different side-effect profile. For one thing, it may act as a natural diuretic, which helps reduce fluid retention, one of the major frustrations and source of side effects of synthetic progestins.

The use of unopposed progesterone, even the "natural" form, can shut down your body's production of both estrogen and progesterone by causing you not to ovulate, thus reducing estrogen and progesterone levels normally made by the ovary.[24] Progesterone can also saturate both progesterone and estrogen receptor-binding sites, thereby reducing their receptivity to further action. It must be remembered that progestogens, even "natural" ones, are not without side effects. The impetus to use progesterone creams alone appears to stem more from the fear of estrogen than the superiority or effectiveness of progesterone.

In truth, "natural" is a matter of degree. The body cannot convert a plant steroid into a human steroid. In order to be bioavailable and bioactive, that is, in a form the body can use, even the wild Mexican yam *(Dioscorea villosa)* from which natural progesterone is often derived, must be altered in a laboratory. The molecular components of wild yam are called "precursor molecules" because they can act as building blocks for other substances, like estrogen and progesterone.[25] The majority of wild yam creams, as well as most natural progesterone, are derived primarily from soybeans. Many products use the name "Mexican yam" because of its healthful reputation. All the natural progesterone produced by the three main manufacturers (Upjohn, Berlichem, and Diosynth) comes from soybeans.

While synthetic progestins are not exact duplicates of the progesterone made by a woman's body and may interact with the body differently on a cellular level, neither is "natural" progesterone an exact duplicate. After processing in the lab, however, "natural" progesterone is molecularly very close. Despite some organic manufacturers' claims, there are no known enzymatic pathways that exist to change yams that we eat or tincture of yam into a usable hormone. Therefore wild yam products that do not contain USP–grade natural progesterone (the converted form that makes it bioavailable) cannot be used by the body. Studies indicate that micronized progesterone combined with olive oil is better than that in peanut oil, which is less expensive and most common.

In other words, many of the yam creams sold in natural food stores and over the Internet are worthless. Many do not contain USP-grade natural progesterone and/or they vary considerably in the amount of usable hormone they do contain. The result is that some women are living with false hope of boosting their health, while others are being under- or overdosed with progesterone. To escape FDA regulations, natural progesterone is frequently sold as a cosmetic or face cream, rather than as hormonal replacement. Most women find the idea of a cream appealing, for it conveys a sense of nurturing like a refreshing and soothing lotion instead of a medicine. Whether the product is purchased at the health food store or in a pharmacy, you must remember that phytosterols are still powerful hormones that must be monitored carefully.

The scientific community is only now beginning to include natural progesterone in its studies. Since it cannot be patented, large drug companies have shown little interest in promoting it. Our local pharmacist enjoys and knows how to compound pure, fresh ingredients in accurate doses. When we use natural progesterone at A Woman's Place, he has shown remarkable flexibility in making adjustments in prescriptions to find the right balance for the individual woman (Dollar Drug, 1-800-728-3173, free shipping within the continental United States). Or we refer patients to the Women's International Pharmacy (1-800-279-5708).

While natural progesterone appears to reduce the side effects found with synthetic progestins, some still remain. The most common complaint is sedation. It is best taken at night or in two smaller doses, morning and night. There are always unique individual responses. Kathi found, for example, that natural progesterone caused her to produce large amounts of gas and have colicky stomach pains. Brenda suffered severe depression until it was discovered the yam cream she had been slathering on contained high doses of progesterone and her blood level was severely elevated. Women who are especially sensitive to the side effects of synthetic progestins may or may not find relief with natural progesterone. The typical progesterone pattern of mood swings, headaches, and breakthrough bleeding can still occur.

How to Take Micronized (Natural) Progesterone

As a cream, apply it to an area of thin soft skin such as chest, breasts, lower abdomen, inner thighs, wrists, inner arms, or neck. Since areas can become saturated, you are advised to rotate areas of application. We don't recommend using it on the face. The cream is absorbed into the fatty layer under the skin and is transferred to the bloodstream, bypassing the digestive system and liver, and circulated to progesterone receptor sites throughout the body. For some women, natural progesterone cream very effectively relieves menopausal symptoms but it does not regulate periods or provide proven cardiovascular or osteoporotic protection. Many women prefer it because they can make slight adjustments as needed. However, its inexactness is a major drawback. Typical instructions for use and dose include:

1. Try rubbing on ¼ teaspoon twice a day from day 7 to day 21 of a typical 28-day cycle.
2. ½ teaspoon is recommended day 21 to day 1 of the period.
3. Do not use it during the period itself.
4. If there is no period, this schedule can be based on a calendar.
5. For vaginal dryness, ¼ to ½ teaspoon a day can be inserted directly into the vagina.
6. For hot flashes, some women find better control by using ½ teaspoon throughout the cycle and by adding natural estrogen.

Lozenges have the advantage of more precise dosage as well as direct absorption into the bloodstream within three to five minutes. Because they are by prescription, you can be confident about purity, quality, and dose. The oil added to make natural progesterone bioavailable can leave a residue in the mouth that some women find distasteful.

Capsules are precise and convenient. Twenty-five to 50 milligrams is recommended for continuous therapy or 300 milligrams for fourteen days, with 200 milligrams taken at night and 100 milligrams taken in the morning.

Think about it . . .
"Forget the fountain of youth. We have the cream." This could easily be the rallying call for a great number of women who are convinced more conventional therapy is not for them. While there is something laudable about becoming healthy in as natural a way as possible, the criteria for "natural" are not measured by using something that can be rubbed on, brewed, or obtained without a prescription. When a friend tells you about "the latest and greatest," what are your criteria for evaluation? Is word of mouth enough? . . . finding it on the Internet? . . . discovering most doctors are against it? Do your choices focus on symptom relief or your overall, long-term health and risk patterns?

No practitioner, at this time, has proof that natural progesterone and phytoestrogens, while relieving symptoms of menopause, also provide the same protective effect of the more traditional forms of therapy. The most definitive evidence to date is the PEPI Trial's use of natural oral progesterone and estrogen, demonstrating its cardiovascular protection. In fact it was the only combination of estrogen and progesterone that elevated the HDL.

Preliminary studies do suggest, however, that these "alternative" medicines will increase the choices that women have for symptom relief and possible reduction of cardiovascular and osteoporotic risk, and pharmacological preference. Unfortunately it is the rare insurance plan that includes them on their formularies, meaning out-of-pocket expense for women who, because of higher risk of breast cancer or their personal comfort level, choose something "weaker than a medicine, stronger than a botanical."

Pearls of wisdom about hormone replacement . . .

1. Hormone replacement has its place and time.
2. Hormones cannot be counted on to remove all symptoms of menopause.
3. The decision to use hormone replacement therapy should primarily be a consideration of risk factors rather than symptomatic relief.
4. Botanicals cannot remove risks to the same degree that hormone replacement therapy can.
5. Generic brands of hormones are not always a good choice and may not give you the same relief and/or side effect profile as the pharmaceutical brand. Make sure your pharmacist does not switch to generic without informing you.
6. Lifestyle choices are helpful alone or as an adjunct in reducing risk factors for the diseases for which estrogen is protective, such as cardiovascular disease, osteoporosis, colon cancer, and diabetes.

LATEST BREAKING NEWS

A recent study on HRT and heart disease could influence your decision about hormone use. The "HERS" study showed that people with existing heart disease should not begin hormone therapy because in the short-term they will not benefit and may be harmed. Such women who are already taking HRT are advised to continue.

Ongoing research indicates the positive benefits of natural progesterone versus synthetic versions for women who are on hormone replacement. It is produced by Solvay pharmaceuticals, and your doctor can write a prescription for it. Solvay also produces a user-friendly estrogen, estratab.

18

Looking at the Bonuses

HORMONES AND COLON CANCER, ALZHEIMER'S DISEASE, AND DIABETES

"Well, Mrs. Wade, your lipid panel is not exactly what I would like to see but it is improving. You're small boned, but your DEXA results indicate your bone density is good. Apparently your love of running has paid off. Whether HRT is the best course for you may be difficult to answer. You are taking good care of yourself and appear to have most symptoms of menopause under control."

Despite her excellent report, Virginia Wade left the doctor's office with a prescription for hormones. Why? Because even though her major risk factors seemed under control, Virginia had additional considerations. Both her father and grandfather had died from colon cancer, and her mother was clearly developing signs of Alzheimer's disease. While estrogen's ability to protect against these two diseases is in need of further research, the link seems to be growing ever stronger.

WHAT DOES COLON CANCER HAVE TO DO WITH MENOPAUSE?

It may surprise you to learn that colon cancer is the second most common cause of death from cancer in the United States.

260

Virginia has good reason to worry, for fifty-one thousand women developed colon cancer in 1995 and one-half will die from the disease and its complications. Recent studies indicate up to a 50 percent reduction in the chance of dying from colon cancer if a woman uses ERT. The greatest reduction in risk for getting colon cancer or surviving it was among those women with longtime estrogen use. Among slender women, risks were lowered by up to 75 percent.[1]

Laboratory experiments have shown that estrogen reduces bile acids, and that reduction lowers the risk of colon cancer. There is some evidence that protection is greatest for current or recent users. Along with hormone replacement, however, a woman's health habits are equally important. The dramatic difference in risk for women who use hormone replacement may also be influenced by the fact that such women are more likely to have health checkups, especially during the crucial forty to sixty age range, than those who have not visited their doctors. Protection also occurs by eating fruits and vegetables, wheat bran cereal, and taking calcium supplements, which also play a role in lowering bile acids.[2] Numerous studies show that taking aspirin or NSAIDS daily lowers risk, although these medications bring their own risks.

AND THEN THERE'S ALZHEIMER'S . . .

"Here, Mother, let me take your purse. I'll carry it for a while." My mother, a frail and tiny version of her former self, handed me what had become her symbol of normalcy and activity. The days when her purse was her passport to life for driving, purchasing, identifying her as the active mother of two, wife of Wilburn, citizen of Texas were long gone. Still, the need for the purse continued, like a trusted companion whom one wouldn't think of leaving behind. While Mother remembered little of the usual routines of life, she never forgot to take her purse, even though she continually forgot where she had put it.

"Mother!" I exclaimed. "What in the world do you have in here? It weighs a ton!" I quickly began a search of the multiple caverns that contained the treasures she had deemed necessary for our venture out. Bolts of Kleenex, a lone lipstick, dental floss, her aqua-rimmed, rhinestone-studded sunglasses, an empty coin purse—and two carefully wrapped sets of spoons!

"Mother, what are you doing with all these spoons in your purse?" I queried, immediately sorry I had asked.

Blushing slightly, she stumbled for an explanation, "Well, you never know when you might need them," she replied defensively. "Besides, Jimmy needs them to stir his martini when we go to dinner."

I thought of Jimmy, the patient, loving physician who had married Mother knowing Alzheimer's disease had already begun to chip away her reality. He had died the year before. Now I was struggling to keep Mother settled in what was to be the first of a series of facilities where she could receive the round-the-clock care she increasingly needed.

Mother's journey with Alzheimer's took almost twenty years. Her decline was slow but steady and my children, my husband, and my life were forever impacted by the experience of watching a perfectly healthy human being slowly lose her mind. Our journey is not over, however, for Dr. Mayo and I now face the much more rapid decline of his mother to the same affliction.

Rapid or slow, Alzheimer's is devastating. While new information is being gathered, there is still no technology for its diagnosis or cure. Recently a genetic link was uncovered—not a pretty thought for Dr. Mayo and myself. A menopausal woman's life is likely to be impacted in two ways by Alzheimer's disease.

1. Protection against Alzheimer's is reduced by declining estrogen levels.
2. A midlife woman is likely to be the caretaker for an aging parent who may have Alzheimer's.

The parent with Alzheimer's is apt to be a woman. Alzheimer's is the most common cause of the loss of mental function, rendering a person incapable of living independently. Rarely occurring in younger people, symptoms may appear around age sixty-five, and the number of new people affected doubles every 4.5

years. By age eighty-five, it is estimated somewhere between 25–50 percent of the population are victims in various stages.

The earliest signs are inability to recall and learn new information. Finding the right word becomes difficult, and eventually disorientation and getting lost occurs. Needless to say, being unable to remember makes one suspicious, depressed, and irritable. When delusions develop, sorting out reality becomes a challenge for the person who is ill as well as for the caregiver.

It is a myth that getting old inevitably means poorer mental functioning. Take heart in the fact that the majority of people age "moderately well" and may deal with only some lack of memory and recall. Ten to thirty percent of aging people avoid disease and maintain high cognitive function and the ability to learn and reason. Even when we respond more slowly, the ability to think is intact and we compensate by adopting different thinking strategies. While the brain's cerebral cortex shrinks by about 10 percent, this is a modest change and does not occur in all parts of the brain.

IS ESTROGEN THE ANSWER FOR ALZHEIMER'S?

The numbers are still small, but studies of estrogen use and Alzheimer's suggest, but so far do not prove, that estrogen is protective.[3] A 1996 study from Columbia University added a new dimension to what is known. Described in a leading British medical journal, estrogen proved equally protective for black, white, and Hispanic women who had taken it for ten years or more.[4] Their chance of developing Alzheimer's was reduced by at least one-third. This is the first study that eliminates the possibility of the results being attributed to a white, upper-middle-class bias.

Studies at Leisure World in Southern California indicate that a 30 percent protective effect of ERT appears to be linked to longer use and dosage.[5] Keep in mind that women who develop Alzheimer's are less likely to have used ERT. We know that in women without dementia, estrogen improves verbal learning, enhances memory, but impacts nonverbal skills to a lesser degree.[6] (Women are more likely than men to lose their ability to remember names of things.) Evidence exists that estrogen may delay symptoms, as well as preventing and moderating their severity.

A review of both open and double-blind placebo-controlled trials was reported at the 1995 North American Menopause Society meeting. Estrogen replacement resulted in significant improvement in memory, especially in verbal ability, compared to untreated patients, even when estrogen was given after the onset of the disease. As observed by the patients' caregivers, improvement occurred in test scores of memory orientation and calculation and in daily living.

The observation that there is a link between weight and Alzheimer's further confirms the role of estrogen. Heavy women, who make estrogen in their fat cells, are less likely to get the disease, even when all other variables are accounted for.[7] Specifically, there was a connection between higher body weight and better naming abilities.

Women who have had a heart attack are five times more likely to develop Alzheimer's. This is not so for men. It is believed that women are more vulnerable after such complicating medical events.[8]

Older women with Alzheimer's have been observed to have lower levels of estrone sulfate. The protective effect of estrogen is most likely due to its ability to increase blood flow and modify cellular processes. There are estrogen receptors in the central nervous system. Estrogen increases projections and synapses between neurons. Investigation of Premarin and one of its components, equilin—an ingredient not found in other estrogens—has been shown to more effectively stimulate the growth of neurons in the frontal, temporal, and occipital regions of the brain. Maintenance of neurons is essential for good brain function, and women whose genetic risk for Alzheimer's is high should seriously consider Premarin.

Evidence exists that neurons are damaged by what is called "oxidative stress," resulting from the great increase in free radicals (unattached oxygen pieces) that comes as we age. Amyloid proteins, believed to be the source of the amyloid plaques found in the brain of those with Alzheimer's disease, set in motion the mechanism of producing free radicals. Estrogen does act as an antioxidant. This additionally explains why studies have shown high doses of vitamin E, which is also an antioxidant, to be effective in improving function of those with Alzheimer's.

Inflammation of the brain is another contributor to Alzheimer's that can result in a one-thousand–fold increase in amyloid protein. Inflammation is due to physical and psychological stressors (toxins from within and without the body, diet, infections, or the imbalance of various enzymatic and nonenzymatic antioxidant defense systems). The chemical process involved results in cell death. Consequently there has been much in the news suggesting people at risk take anti-inflammatory drugs.

WHY NOT SOME OTHER MEDICINE JUST FOR ALZHEIMER'S?

There are now two medications approved for treatment of Alzheimer's, Tacrine and Aricept. The success of their use is modest. So what can you do to protect yourself? Studies suggest that impaired brain function is a result of disease, not age. This means that, barring disease, continuing to challenge the brain can improve its function. Like the rest of your body, the brain needs exercise. "Working out" your brain results in neurons sprouting dendrites, which increases the paths of communication between cells. Those who keep active, are open to new experiences, reduce stress, maintain a sense of control, and are involved with others are more likely to do well as they age.

For the curious . . . Acetylcholine is the most important neurotransmitter for memory and cognitive function. Estrogen may influence the enzyme involved in synthesis of acetylcholine.

While we would not recommend daily use of traditional anti-inflammatory medications because of the risk to the gastrointestinal tract and the far-reaching negative health effects, natural supplements seem in order. Increasing knowledge of the chemistry of the disease makes daily use of B12 (100–1000 mg), B6

(1–100 mg), folate (1–20 mg), and betaine (1–3 grams) good choices. The anti-inflammatory properties of turmeric and ginger are better choices than aspirin or NSAIDS. Depending on personal risk factors and history, consideration of a conjugated estrogen, like Premarin, with its equilin component, should be considered for maximum protection.

DIABETES AND ESTROGEN

Diabetes is a disease in which there is a high level of glucose (sugar) in the blood that does not pass into the cells for use as an energy source. This leaves cells starving for food, and over time may cause other diseases of the eyes, kidneys, nerves, or heart. The goal of treatment is to improve or maintain healthy blood glucose levels. Type I diabetics are likely to experience menopause at an early age (the average is at age forty-two, as opposed to age fifty for the general population).[9]

Diabetic control for some, but not all diabetics, is maintained by eating a balanced low-glycemic, high-fiber diet (see chapter 13), exercising, and keeping a healthy weight. As we age, most people have more difficulty controlling their blood sugar and many develop insulin resistance, a condition in which the cells simply ignore the insulin sent to lower the blood sugar—diabetics experience even more trouble. It is here that estrogen plays its role, for it is known to improve the regulation of blood sugar. But perhaps more important, it is protective against the cardiovascular problems diabetics often face.

Since progestins affect carbohydrate metabolism, they are given with caution to diabetic women, thus preventing most of them from using birth control pills. At menopause natural progesterone is least likely to cause hyperinsulinemia. Today many doctors dismiss the progesterone effect as small enough to warrant its use. Careful monitoring for individual response is always in order. To prevent complications and monitor progress, diabetic women should be tested every three to four months, using a glycosylated hemoglobin test (HemA1C). This would give an accurate view of blood sugar levels over longer periods of time, a more exact way to monitor blood sugar than previous tests

monitoring fasting blood glucose levels or the three-hour glucose tolerance test.

Pearls of wisdom for three serious diseases . . .

1. Sound nutrition can prevent the expression of disease and/or
   moderate its expression.
2. Stay active mentally and physically.
3. Master stress-reduction techniques.

19

Checking Out the Fine Print

FACING THE RISKS OF BREAST CANCER

"Say, Doreen, have you followed up on the lump Dr. Rosalie found?" I asked my friend during one of our periodic long-distance catch-up sessions.

"Mary Ann, I have been so swamped, I haven't been in . . . I'll do it, I'll do it," she promised. Somehow another month passed, and when she called her doctor, he suggested that "maybe" she should come in for a biopsy. That "maybe" provided just enough excuse not to make an immediate appointment.

Finally, during a brief visit to our area, we literally deposited her in the office of our local breast cancer expert. His report had no "maybe" about it. The presentation and size of her lump convinced him, even without a biopsy, that she was most likely dealing with a cancer. He referred her directly to a large cancer institute. And sadly, he was right. She had been waiting for the lump to magically disappear, when it actually was a tumor containing two of the most virulent, rapidly growing varieties of breast cancer around. By the time two years had passed, her procrastination had cost Doreen her life.

An expert would have picked Doreen as someone with a high risk for breast cancer because of the number of her risk factors. Her one child was adopted, she had suffered a miscarriage, she was overweight, and her diet included lots of fast foods. As she

For the curious . . .
- Sixty out of every one hundred patients with breast cancer require treatment that involves mastectomy or breast-conserving surgery with radiotherapy.
- Out of every fifty-six American women, twenty-eight can expect to die from heart disease, eight will develop osteoporosis, and seven will develop breast cancer.

obtained increasing success professionally, there had been plenty of stress, but no time for exercise.

Doreen was not unlike 20–25 percent of women who wait at least two to three months before seeking medical care after finding a breast lump or other cancer sign or symptom.[1] They convince themselves the lump is nothing serious and if they react, they'll look like an alarmist. Most people have a desire to feel in control of their health and try to avoid medical procedures that might cause disruption in their routine. In fact, as with Doreen, the desire not to take time from work is the number one reason given for delay in seeking medical evaluation, followed by family and other commitments.

Our pattern as women of taking care of everyone and everything sometimes impacts our own health. In the case of breast cancer, the delay can be deadly. What you are fearful about determines your action. The underlying fear of cancer, anxiety about losing a breast and/or having surgery, tends to immobilize a woman. Fortunately anxiety stemming from wanting to know usually results in making an appointment to see a doctor and achieving resolution. While not all breast cancers are alike, premenopausal breast cancer is generally more aggressive. Early detection is critical.

Factors Related to the Risk of Breast Cancer

Decreases Risk	Increases Risk
Late first period (age 16)	Early first period (ages 10–12)
Birth of first child when in twenties	Birth of first child after age 30
Greater number of children	Few or one child*
Breast-feeding	Not breast-feeding
Being a vegetarian	Eating high fat/meat-based diet**
Exercise***	Sedentary lifestyle
Healthy weight	Being overweight
Full-term pregnancy	Having miscarriage/abortion
Surgical menopause	Going through regular menopause
No family history	Family history among young women on maternal side****
Early menopause (before age 45)	Late menopause (after age 51)

*Observational studies show that women who do not ovulate regularly and those who are infertile, therefore exposed to less progesterone, have an increased risk of breast cancer later in life. Women athletes and those suffering from anorexia would fall into this category. A reduction in the total number of menstrual cycles during life, such as in full-term pregnancy, reduces risk.[2]

**A 1996 Italian study, however, reported a greater connection between starch and breast cancer than between fat and breast cancer. Women were 39 percent more likely to develop breast cancer if their diet was high in starch versus a low-starch diet.[3]

***Among premenopausal women, exercise lowers breast cancer. After menopause the results are more conflicting. Two of the most recent and well-done studies demonstrated a reduced risk with just recreational physical activity. Being active, not a great athlete, is the key.

****The increased risk is more for premenopausal breast cancer rather than postmenopausal.[4] Early breast cancer tends to be more genetic in origin and likely to be passed on.

HOW LIKELY AM I TO GET BREAST CANCER?

If she lives to age eighty, every woman has a lifetime risk of 1 in 9 of getting breast cancer. For women who have given birth, risks are 1 in 222 up to age thirty-nine, 1 in 26 from age forty to fifty-nine, and 1 in 15 from age sixty to seventy-nine.[5] The absolute risk of a typical fifty-year-old developing breast cancer over the next thirty years is 9 percent. Increase that risk by 30 percent for HRT use, and absolute risk increases to 12 percent.[6] These sta-

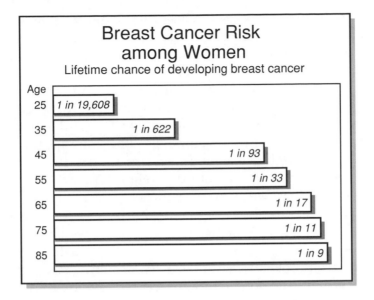

Breast Cancer Risk among Women

Lifetime chance of developing breast cancer

Age	
25	1 in 19,608
35	1 in 622
45	1 in 93
55	1 in 33
65	1 in 17
75	1 in 11
85	1 in 9

tistical odds, however, are for the population as a whole. Your risk depends on your particular health history.

Over the last four decades the risk has increased, leveling out in 1987. A surge occurred in the early 1980s when new technology increased the ability to more accurately identify small tumors. The number of people actually dying has stayed about the same, around forty-six thousand a year. So despite more people getting breast cancer, the death rate has actually gone down. The five-year survival rate has risen from 78 percent in 1940 to 93 percent in 1993. Thanks to (1) earlier diagnosis, (2) increased use of mammography, and (3) improved treatment options, 50–75 percent of women are being cured.

Whatever your personal risk factors are, the fear of breast cancer remains the major reason expressed for not considering hormone replacement. And yet many women don't make even the most rudimentary effort to protect themselves—by self-examinations. The truth is, depending on the type of doctor you visit, if you don't examine your breasts, they may not be examined. If you are between fifty and seventy-five years old and make routine visits to a gynecologist, there is a 90 percent chance he or she will do a breast exam—57 percent of internists and 40 percent of family doctors include this routine service. Even diligent self-examination cannot pick up the minute lesions that can be seen on a mammogram. The mammogram remains the only statistically significant procedure known to affect mortality.

Although no one knows the exact formula for what causes breast cancer, we are beginning to understand some of the things that influence its development. For example, the *Lancet* reports that higher weight infants are more likely to later develop breast cancer than lower weight infants. This leads to speculation that, for some, the mechanism for breast cancer begins in the womb.[7] The newest information concerns the impact of exercise. Whether it is the loss of weight that often occurs with exercise or the exercise itself that lowers breast cancer risk is not clear. The most precise picture has come from a Norwegian study of more than twenty-five thousand women. Even after adjusting for age, body mass, dietary intake, and number of children, women who exercised were at significantly less risk.[8] Another preventative step available to anyone is modification of diet to include more soy, flaxseed oil, and other essential oils (see chapter 13).

New technology that can identify a breast cancer gene helps put the concept of risk factors that are under our control into better perspective. Around 25 percent of breast cancer has a genetic basis, meaning 75 percent is influenced by other factors. Only 5–10 percent of women have the gene for breast cancer. A sampling of families in which there is a history of breast cancer indicates those who carry the gene have a 19 percent chance of developing breast cancer by age forty and an 85 percent chance by the time they reach age eighty-five.[9] A survey of the general population who carry the gene gives a little more hope, placing the risk for an eighty-five-year-old woman at 56 percent.[10] A consensus statement published by the *Journal of the American Medical Association* (vol. 277, 1997, pages 997–1003) advises women who carry the BRAC1 or BRAC2 gene to begin self-exams at age eighteen and have a clinical breast exam or mammogram once or twice a year beginning between the ages of twenty-five to thirty-five.

For the curious . . .
Who will or will not develop breast cancer is not just the luck of the draw, but a combination of factors that increases or decreases a person's chance of becoming ill. As you observed when you read the factors that affect risk, many of them are within an individual's control, so you do have some control over the risk factors. From a statistical point of view, risk is a numerical measure of how likely any woman is to become ill. It is important that you grasp the concept of relative risk (RR) in order to understand how different health interventions or exposures will affect your actual risk of getting breast cancer.

Relative risk is the chance one group, who is alike in certain ways (fifty-year-old exercisers, for example), versus another group, who is alike in different ways (fifty-year-old couch potatoes), have of getting a disease. When a study speaks of a relative risk above 2.0, it means the variable that is being measured—breast cancer—is meaningfully affected by whatever the difference is. In our example, if the relative risk was 2.1, for instance, it would say that being a couch potato is likely to increase the odds of your getting breast cancer. RRs below or up to 2.0 are considered weak associations and may be due to chance.

An important thing to note is an increase of RR from 1.0, which says there is no risk, to a RR of 1.5 can be stated as a 50 percent increase in risk. News headlines then blare, for example, that being "a couch potato increases breast cancer by 50 percent"—which, while technically correct, does not convey an accurate personal risk for that individual. It certainly doesn't mean that any woman who doesn't exercise has a 50 percent chance of breast cancer. It does mean that whatever her risk (1 in 9 for a lifetime risk for the general population), not exercising might increase it slightly.

Since carrying the genes also increases the odds of ovarian and colorectal cancer, screening for them is advised.

A high family risk motivates some women to reduce their personal risk by having their breasts removed before cancer strikes. A seventeen-year study from The Mayo Clinic revealed a 91 percent reduction in cancer for women whose family or medical history indicated they were likely to develop the disease and who had their breasts removed.[11]

Estrogen and Breast Cancer

Breast cancer is closing in on lung cancer as the most common cancer in women, with an estimated incidence of 182,000 in 1995. The fact that it is over two hundred times more common in women than men is strongly suggestive of some hormonal involvement. Even after menopause, when a woman's body is in a state of estrogen deficiency compared to her premenopausal days, breast cancer continues to rise. The biggest increase in breast cancer is among sixty-five- to eighty-five-year-olds. Many women of this age never used hormones or if they did, they used estrogen only.

It should be noted that the vast majority of women who have taken birth control pills have not developed breast cancer. This is even the case with the new low-dose variety, which still has four times the estrogen found in the typical hormone replacement dosages. Neither do the high hormones of pregnancy influence breast cancer. The few differences in prognosis that appear in some studies have been attributed to late diagnosis, not to increased susceptibility.

Obviously the particular role estrogen plays in breast cancer is multifaceted and complex. Looking closely at the factors that increase and decrease the odds of getting breast cancer, one thing becomes very clear. The total exposure of a woman to estrogen—particularly in relation to the number of menstrual cycles she has had in her lifetime—her progesterone production, and the number of ovulation cycles are ingredients in the breast cancer recipe.

Concern over estrogen arises from the fact that in the laboratory estrogen has been shown to increase the rate of cell division (mitosis) in breast cells, whereas substances like tamoxifen, and continuous progestogens, reduce cell division. The significance of all this is that increased cell division is a characteristic of cancer.

Because the breast has the capacity to amass estrogen within the fluid that resides in the ductal structures of the breast, concentrations of estrogen can be ten- to fortyfold greater than in the bloodstream. Although estrogen blood levels drop at menopause, breast-fluid estrogen remains at very high levels. In fact even without estrogen replacement, the estrogen in the breast ducts of premenopausal and postmenopausal women is higher than normally found in blood at the midcycle peak. When estrogen replacement is given, both blood and ductal fluid estrogen levels rise even higher.

The body's ability to concentrate estrogen in the breast more than in the lining of the uterus may account for why the breast cancer rate continues to go up with age while the uterine cancer rate does not. It has been observed that fat cells, which have the ability to convert androgens into estrone and estradiol throughout the body, are particularly adept at doing their job in breast tissue adjacent to a carcinoma.[12]

IF ESTROGEN CAN BE A BAD GUY, IS PROGESTERONE THE GOOD GUY?

Your fat cells' ability to change androgens into estrogens can be tempered or blocked by progesterone—at least this has been shown in the laboratory. Progesterone is known to suppress some of the growth factors that are responsible for increasing mitosis and mutations. It also plays a part in converting the strongest form of estrogen—estradiol—into its weaker forms—estrone and estriol.

Before menopause, progesterone, like estrogen, concentrates in breast ductal fluid in amounts higher than that found in the blood. So far there is no proof that the postmenopausal breast selectively concentrates progesterone as it did prior to menopause. Therefore scientists speculate that a menopausal woman's

For the curious . . .
Breast adipose tissue (fat) contains the aromatase enzyme necessary for androgen conversion. Progesterone decreases aromatase activity in the endometrium and in breast cancer cells in vitro. Another function of progesterone is to increase the activity of estradiol dehydrogenase, an enzyme that changes estrogen into its weaker metabolites.

breast tissue may be exposed to very high levels of unopposed estrogen, and that the lower annual breast cancer incidence before menopause may be in part due to the local presence of progesterone.[13] Progesterone production is fairly stable by age fifteen and begins to decline around age thirty-five.[14]

A WORD ABOUT RECEPTORS

Progesterone may also protect against breast cancer because it reduces the number of estradiol receptors. A receptor is like a designated parking space. Estradiol receptors are very particular about allowing anything but estradiol into its space. Once parked, receptors are activated by the hormone so they can accomplish their work in the body. Besides specific spaces for estrogen, there are parking spots reserved for progesterone.

These designated receptors (parking spaces) for estrogen and progesterone are found most abundantly in the uterus and breast. By reducing the number of parking spaces for estradiol, progesterone lessens its overall impact. It is important to note that progesterone also reduces the production of its own receptors.[15] The consequence is an undermining of its protective effect on the breast cells, especially if unopposed progesterone is administered. The use of an intermittent or continuous estrogenic substance is essential to maintain the production of progesterone receptors.

The presence of both estrogen and progesterone receptors has been noted in women with less aggressive forms of breast cancer. After prolonged treatment, in virtually all advanced breast cancers, resistance to hormones develops. The exact role of progesterone and antiprogesterone functions are among the most complex of all steroid hormones, perhaps because there are two natural forms of progesterone that act differently.

IF ESTROGEN IS RELATED TO BREAST CANCER, WHY SHOULD ANYONE TAKE IT?

Flooding your body with more estrogen than it needs to keep you functioning and healthy should not be anyone's agenda. On the other hand, a precise replacement of estrogen may be essential for some women to feel healthy because it can give protection against their unique risk factors. While estrogen's role in breast cancer is important and should be seriously considered, other risk factors must be added to the mix to determine each individual's particular susceptibility. *Breast cancer is not caused by estrogen acting alone, but by a multitude of factors that combine to overcome a woman's immune system, making her vulnerable to illness.* What follows is a brief synopsis of what is currently reported about the interplay of estrogen and breast cancer in peer-reviewed journals.

It may surprise you to learn that over fifty studies have been conducted on breast cancer and estrogen. The results are mixed. Most have not shown an effect. Some say estrogen decreases cancer. Some say that it increases your odds of breast cancer.[16] It should be noted that the majority of studies showing an increase in breast cancers are from Europe, where stronger doses of estrogen are used.

A 1997 recommendation of the *Journal of the American Medical Association* states that if you have a high heart attack risk and *one* close relative with breast cancer, the benefits of HRT outweigh the risks. If you have no heart disease or osteoporotic risk factors and *two* close relatives with breast cancer, don't take HRT.[17]

277

ESTROGEN MAY RESULT IN A SLIGHT INCREASE IN BREAST CANCER

Some studies that looked at daily or less use for over ten years indicate a slight increase in breast cancer. Unopposed estrogen means a woman does not take any progestins or progesterone. Remember that a relative risk of 1 means no risk and 2 means a risk not due to chance. A Swedish study, which used a small group of several hundred women but extrapolated their results to 23,244 women, found an increase of breast cancer in post-menopausal women of RR 1.1 for short-term use and RR 1.7 after nine years of use.[18] The women had taken estradiol at a strength of 1.25 milligrams.

No risk was discovered for those using the conjugated estrogen premarin, which contains all three varieties of estrogen—estradiol, estrone, and estriol. While this study is frequently quoted, its scientific validity is regularly criticized.[19] Research done on 121,700 nurses indicated a 46 percent increase in risk of death from breast cancer among current estrogen users.[20] This was an increased relative risk of 1.46 for women currently on estrogen replacement, and was widely reported in the newspapers with headlines declaring an almost 50 percent increase in breast cancer among estrogen users.

To put this in perspective—if one hundred women aged fifty were monitored for the next twenty years, five would develop breast cancer by the age of seventy. If these same women had been given unopposed estrogen, and their risk increased by 40 percent, it would mean two extra women, a total of seven, would develop breast cancer.

OR MAYBE NOT . . .

The Harvard Nurses' Health Study quoted above has sixteen years of follow-up (1976–1992). Although it found an increased risk for current users of hormones, it also stated that women who had previously used estrogen, even for as long as ten or more years, were not at increased risk. Such seeming discrepancies point out the complexity of the interactions involved in developing breast cancer and the importance of paying attention to the multitude of risk factors for breast cancer.

The Cancer Society's Cancer Prevention Study II, involving 422,373 postmenopausal women, is considerably larger than the Nurses' Health Study. It has also shattered previous beliefs about hormone replacement and breast cancer. The postmenopausal women in their study were found to have a better prognosis if they had taken hormone replacement (HRT) before their diagnosis.[21] Women who have ever taken estrogen replacement are 16 percent less likely to die of breast cancer than nonusers.[22] Women who started hormone replacement before forty were least likely to die from their breast cancer and had a 34 percent decrease in risk. In general, estrogen users were 20 percent less likely to die of the disease, perhaps because they reduced the possibility of developing more aggressive forms of breast cancer and contracting the slow-growing variety. In this large study, long-term use of more than ten years did not increase risk of dying from breast cancer.

In 1989 follow-up and reevaluation of 10,366 consecutive benign breast cancer biopsy specimens collected between 1950 and 1968 provided the basis for calculating relative risk for a variety of variables. The relative risk of developing breast cancer for women who used estrogen was RR 0.98 versus RR 1.8 for those who did not.[23] Studies using Premarin, the most commonly prescribed estrogen replacement, have found no meaningful increased risk of breast cancer with the standard doses when taken for less than ten years.[24]

A few studies have shown continual use of estrogen and progesterone reduced risk of breast cancer.[25] Estrogen may actually be protective. Women on birth control pills or estrogen replacement have been found to have lower grade, smaller size cancers, with less metastases (spread) and with a more favorable prognosis, when compared with age-matched breast cancer patients not on hormones.[26] Five hundred thirty-seven women with breast cancer were compared to 492 randomly selected women without breast cancer, and no difference in risk due to estrogen was found, even though about 60 percent had used hormone therapy.[27]

279

The combination of estrogen and progesterone is confirmed to provide even greater protection for two reasons: (1) they enhance the immune system and (2) they maintain a healthy balance of hormonal receptors.[28] Estrogen stimulates production of its own receptors and those of progesterone. Left unopposed, estrogen will increase its own receptors. But when progesterone is added, the estrogen effect is counteracted, even though excess progesterone ultimately decreases the number of its own receptors.

Progesterone's role in maintaining healthy breast tissue may lie in its ability to maintain hormonal balance in breast tissue. After ovulation ceases, the progesterone receptors become less functional. The thirty to forty years left in a woman's life is lived with estrogen dominance in the breast tissue. Despite this, not everyone develops hormonally related breast cancer. Other forms of breast cancers may be driven by genetic and other factors, quite apart from hormones.

If you need to use estrogen because of personal risk factors—heart disease, osteoporosis, or Alzheimer's disease—taking a combination of hormones (estrogen and progesterone) may ultimately be the best replacement when considering breast cancer risk. This is true even after a hysterectomy, when progesterone's protection against uterine cancer is not needed. Use of the less potent forms of estrogen—estrone and estriol—or a hormonal combination, and perhaps natural rather than synthetic products, should be considered, especially when family history or other factors increase your risk.

For their high-risk patients, many natural practitioners recommend estriol, the weakest estrogen and the one version thought to be most protective against cancer (see chapter 17). Like cholesterol, hormones all have good and bad effects determined by their appropriate balance.

THROW THEM ALL TOGETHER AND WHAT DO YOU HAVE?—META-ANALYSIS

As of 1996 there have been five meta-analysis studies of breast cancer and estrogen use. A meta-analysis is a mathematical tool that combines the results of divergent and sometimes small studies to see if statistically sound results can be seen using the larger combined data. None of the five meta-analyses, combining seventeen studies comparing the relative risk of breast cancer for any woman who has ever used estrogen replacement versus women who have never used it, shows an increase in the relative risk of breast cancer for women taking hormones.[29]

Five of the longest studies, over fifteen years, showed a relative risk from 1.04–1.14. No difference was seen with the addition of progesterone. Researchers also compared different ways people used hormones, finding a range of relative risk from 1.0–1.07. It appeared that no specific dose or regime proved significantly better or worse than another. Synthetic estrogens may be associated with slightly higher risks than conjugated estrogens (combinations of the three estrogens as found in Premarin and some of the compounded natural estrogens).

Women who were currently using hormones had an increased relative risk from 1.23–1.40. This disappeared if hormones were discontinued as little as two years earlier. In one meta-analysis, the slight increase of breast cancer with current estrogen use was determined to be a very weak association and may be due to the number of current users in that group. At this point, whether the slightly increased risk of breast cancer with long duration (over five years of use) is detection bias or real is unclear and unanswered from the meta-analysis. It must be remembered in all studies that patients who take hormone replacement are different from those who don't because they tend to have more regular medical care and their cancers are more likely to be detected.

CHOOSING HRT AFTER BREAST CANCER

The concern over whether estrogen contributes to breast cancer takes on new meaning when a woman who has had breast cancer is suffering severe menopausal symptoms. These symptoms may not be responsive to other treatments, or the woman may be at high risk for heart disease and/or osteoporosis. Universally, women are asked to discontinue estrogen replacement once a diagnosis of breast cancer is made. After analysis of the specific type of tumor, appropriate treatment, follow-up, and recovery are complete, the issue of whether to again take hormone replacement frequently arises. The 1994 committee opinion from the College of Obstetricians and Gynecologists states that ERT may be considered as a treatment option.

The question becomes more urgent because some of the treatments for breast cancer can trigger a rapid and perhaps premature menopause. The sudden onslaught of signs and symptoms of menopause, along with the effort devoted to recovery, can be overwhelming. Before an appropriate decision is made, several considerations must be taken into account. Is the woman dealing with a lower-risk cancer? Was it detected early? Is it estrogen sensitive? What is the status of axillary lymph nodes and estrogen receptors? What is the size and type of tumor? How much time has elapsed since diagnosis and treatment? In the past, when she consulted with her physician about HRT, the answer was a resounding no. Today, it is maybe.

As we noted, some studies have shown longer survival in breast cancer cases that have occurred while the women were on estrogen.[30] Other studies have found lower incidences of recurrence and longer survival in women given low-dose estrogen replacement after being diagnosed and treated for breast cancer.[31]

The largest and longest case-controlled study of continuous combined estrogen-progesterone therapy given to breast cancer survivors was completed in 1995. It reported no deaths and less recurrence (7 percent) in the estrogen-progesterone users than in matched controls (17 percent). Among progesterone-only users, there was only one recurrence (3 percent), compared to 15 percent of non-progesterone controls. Eighteen percent of the women had a recurrence or developed a cancer in the other breast, yet only 4 percent had used either estrogen-progesterone or progesterone alone. The authors concluded that previous and current estrogen was protective.[32]

Another study, designed to carefully monitor women for breast cancer recurrence, compared one group of women given hormone replacement, both estrogen and progesterone, with another that took no hormones. After six years, no woman had died in the hormone replacement group, whereas 6 percent of the controls had died. Recurrence occurred in six women on HRT and in thirty of those without.

The same researchers noted that a group of women who received progesterone therapy only had no deaths and one recurrence, whereas ten controls in the group who took no hormone died and eighteen had a recurrence. Further evidence that hormone replacement can slow growth of breast cancer came from special monitoring of chemical markers that indicate when recurrence is likely, even though it hasn't occurred yet. On the basis of their increased likelihood to have a recurrence, some women were given progesterone and another matched group was not. Those who received progesterone didn't develop a tumor for twenty-four months, whereas the control group not receiving the hormone developed tumors within four months.[33] Considering all of their results, the researchers concluded that "women taking estrogen with medium-high-dose progesterone do not suffer any disadvantage in respect to their breast cancer and possibly may have a survival advantage over women not taking it."[34]

WHY DO WE SEEM TO BE SEEING MORE BREAST CANCER?

No one really knows why there seems to be an increase in the number of breast cancers diagnosed, but the answer could tie in with those "designated parking spaces" or hormonal receptors located in great numbers in the breast and uterus. As you have probably experienced, even if you have a parking space reserved just for you, occasionally someone else has the audacity to park in it. The same thing happens within our body. While not every chemical that comes along will fit into an estrogen receptor (parking space), there are a few models that do.

Currently we are exposed to about one hundred thousand foreign chemicals, called xenobiotics. They include drugs, pesticides, environmental pollutants, industrial chemicals, and food additives. Many won't fit in an estrogen-specific receptor, but some, the molecular structure of which is similar to estrogen, make themselves right at home. The classic pesticide DDT is one. Yes, DDT has been banned for years, but it bears repeating that DDT and other similar environmental pesticides are still prevalent in our soil and imported in food grown on foreign soils. Carcinogenic exposure, particularly between the ages when a girl begins her period (menarche) and the age when she has her first child, makes her especially vulnerable. High breast-cell turnover, stimulated by high estrogen levels, makes the breast vulnerable, adding to other risk factors that may operate through an estrogen pathway.

I LEFT MY HEALTH IN SAN FRANCISCO

San Francisco has the highest breast cancer rates in the world. On the whole, San Franciscans eat and have access to fresh and healthy foods. Smog is not much of a problem either, but there is always suspicion of an environmental toxin. Other risk factors are also evident. The percentage of single and married career women is high. These women tend to have fewer or no children and when they do become pregnant, they are apt to be older first-time mothers. As a result, fewer have breast-fed or carried full-term pregnancies.

A San Franciscan woman probably lives with the stress of an urban community, perhaps a commute, and has a tension-filled job. And it may be there is simply a genetic pool imparting a higher risk for breast cancer. The fact that San Francisco's women tend to be well-educated and more likely to have medical insurance translates into an educated consumer, who is more likely to make regular trips to her physician, where breast cancer is apt to be discovered.

Obviously there is no proof of exactly what has caused the rise in breast cancer in our lifetime but it appears to be leveling off. We do have some control—our own modifiable risk factors. We can eat less fatty meat, more fruits and vegetables, and more soy products. We can avoid transfatty acids, exercise regularly, build up our immune systems, and schedule our physical exams and mammograms on time.

Pearls of wisdom about breast cancer . . .

1. If you have cancer, you must be a partner with your doctor in your care to ensure your best chance for survival.
2. Depending on your physician, hospital, and which coast you happen to live on, your course of treatment can be radically different from that of other people with the same cancer.
3. Keep up on current research, such as the ongoing Physician's Health Study and Women's Antioxidant Cardiovascular Study, which is testing vitamins C, E, and beta-carotene for their anticancer effects.
4. Any exercise, including recreational physical activity, is protective.
5. Ultrasound is helpful in diagnosing women with dense breasts and high-risk profiles. 3-D displays are helping pick up malignancies.
6. Mammograms reduce the risk of death from breast cancer in women in their forties. Mammography also picks up ductal carcinoma in situ, lesions that are confined to the milk ducts and are more common in younger women. Removing them reduces the risk of invasive cancer recurrence and avoids extensive surgery and other difficult therapies.
7. When surgery is performed during the progestogen (luteal) phase of the menstrual cycle, there is improved survival and a greater recurrence-free interval.[35]
8. Progesterone has been shown to be effective therapy for advanced breast cancer and to reduce intraductal hyperplasia and atypical hyperplasia by 48 percent.[36] Its ability to inhibit mitosis and mutations is the basis on which it is believed to work, although much about progesterone therapy is still theoretical. A French study showed decreased mitosis when progesterone gel was added directly to the breast for thirteen days prior to surgery.
9. Nutritional and herbal supplements that have cellular antioxidant formulas, such as Fem Protect from Metagenics, will aid the body in eliminating toxic free radicals and xenobiotics.

LATEST BREAKING NEWS

The origin of breast cancer continues to be complex and elusive in individual women. The largest study to date indicates that when lean women take a combination of estrogen and progesterone for over five years, their breast cancer risk almost doubles (*JAMA*, 26 January 2000). This means that for every 100,000 women over ages 60 to 64 who are not taking HRT, approximately 350 will develop breast cancer each year. About 400 lean women will develop the disease with over five years' use of estrogen alone, and when progestin is added, the number increases to 560.

Soy research continues to demonstrate the benefits of a phytoestrogen rich diet. Not only does it reduce the risk of breast cancer but it also appears to protect the heart, lower the risk of stroke as effectively as premarin (T. Clark, American Heart Association 38th Annual Conference), and benefit bone.

Part Five

Taking a Closer Look

Things aren't always as they seem. Some physical maladies have symptoms that mimic menopause. When they occur at midlife, they can cause confusion. How can you tell the difference?

Withdrawal of the female hormones—estrogen and progesterone—is the major culprit in menopausal symptomatology. If this were the only thing going on for a woman in midlife, she could expect her experience to be similar to other women her age. But in reality everyone's passage is different. Between 25 and 30 percent of American women have few or no signs of menopause, while the reality of the rest varies from the acknowledgment that their body is acting somewhat differently to near incapacitation.

The reason for the variability is not such a mystery. Genetic propensity, weight, thyroid health, hypoglycemia, stress, PMS, gut and adrenal health, and toxic sensitivities individualize the experience. Our menopause is indeed our own. Nowhere is this more evident than in the ability (or inability) of the adrenal glands to act in reverse synchrony with diminishing ovarian function. The skin, muscle, brain, pineal gland, hair follicles, and body fat work to follow the adrenals' lead in manufacturing and converting necessary hormones. For some women, this is enough, but for those whose overall health has begun to degenerate, menopausal signs and complaints make themselves all too evident. It is best to confront menopause with a focus on total well-being—for some women there is no other choice.

20

Menopause Impostors

Jackie was a busy and impatient lady. "I don't have time to sit and do all these assessments. Just have the doctor give me the pills and I'm out of here," she pleaded to our staff. While we have found that most women want to learn all they can about menopause and the interventions they might be called on to consider, occasionally someone like Jackie appears. Our job remains making her an informed consumer. What Jackie doesn't understand is that other factors besides age and hormones affect the need for and the effectiveness of medication prescribed for menopause.

Take Louise, for example. She was convinced that her lethargy, weight gain, and depression signaled she was perimenopausal. All her friends were and at forty-five she certainly could be. She came into the office prepared to start hormone replacement. Laboratory tests revealed, however, that although she was not yet menopausal, she was suffering from hypothyroidism. Within a month or two, replacement dosage of thyroid left her feeling like her old self.

Ann wasn't sure what was wrong with her. Her nerves were frazzled, her body ached, and she felt hungry much of the time and craved sweets. Several times a day, she would get very shaky and confused. A friend had recommended our clinic, knowing we specialize in midlife health. At fifty-one Ann had eased through the transition into menopause, at least until now.

A thorough history and laboratory tests revealed that most of what Ann was experiencing was related to being hypoglycemic and under severe stress, and not to menopause. While herbs were suggested for her few signs of menopause, like hot flashes, Ann was counseled about changing her eating habits to steady her body's erratic blood sugar levels.

Ann began to practice FREEZE FRAME to reduce stress (see chapter 15), penciled in time for exercise, and agreed to see a counselor for some personal issues that needed resolution. Her progress was slow but one year later, the slim, dynamic, and happy woman who came back for a checkup hardly resembled the frazzled, overweight, and miserable lady we had first met.

Zooey was miserable too. A sixty-year-old former school-teacher, she had been to one doctor after another. Her chart was filled with years of nebulous complaints, all of which added up to frustration and more than once being written off as a "kook" by a perplexed health practitioner. She was tired all the time, suffered aches and pains in most of her joints, was often bloated, and rarely slept through the night. Because of her health risks for osteoporosis and heart disease, she had been taking hormone replacement for several years. At first she blamed the hormones for how bad she felt but after several months of a "hormone holiday" she found they weren't the problem.

Periodically Zooey and her doctor would try a different hormonal brand, mix, or delivery system. Nothing she did seemed to make much difference, and no one seemed to know why. When she was referred to us, Zooey had reluctantly concluded that after all, "she was just getting old" and that there was nothing she could do about her declining health. The usual assessment and history were done and because of the chronic nature of her problems, adrenal stress and gut permeability tests were ordered. Results indicated that Zooey had a gluten intolerance, her adrenal glands were on the verge of burnout, and she suffered from "leaky gut." Remedial measures were instituted and Zooey's life was turned around. Today she is coaching her granddaughter's softball team, has a great outlook on life, and feels anything but old.

Barbara, age forty-six, came to us complaining about her worsening PMS symptoms. Careful diary keeping revealed her "PMS" had spilled over into most of her cycle and was a good indication that she had entered the perimenopause.

These women and countless others like them, remind us of the individual nature of a woman's health and the importance of looking at the big picture before deciding on any one course of action. With other health factors under control, if menopausal interventions are necessary, they can be less potent and are apt to be more effective.

IS IT MENOPAUSE AND/OR SOMETHING ELSE?

The conditions most likely to mask, escalate, or mimic perimenopause or menopause symptoms are the following:

thyroid disorders
hypoglycemia
stress
premenstrual syndrome
adrenal dysfunction
gut permeability

While any of these disorders can affect a woman's quality of life at any age, their incidence increases at midlife.

IT MUST BE YOUR THYROID

Thyroid disease, which includes Hashimoto's thyroiditis—an autoimmune version—is more common in women and increases in midlife. At least 10 percent of women over fifty have thyroid abnormalities. The newest studies estimate that 11 percent of the population have undiagnosed thyroid conditions, up from 5 percent.[1] The presence of other autoimmune diseases or a family history increase your risk. When your body produces either too much thyroid hormone (hyperthyroidism) or too little (hypothyroidism), it can be confused with estrogen deficiency.

Hyperthyroidism, for example, can cause hot flashes, heart palpitations, and insomnia. Hypothyroidism can cause lethargy, memory problems, cold intolerance, and weight gain. The most accurate way to know if you have a thyroid problem is a TSH

291

(thyroid-stimulating hormone) blood test. Be aware that such tests can be affected by illness, stress, and fasting.

If you suffer from hypothyroidism, you may experience swelling around your eyes, dry skin, and sensitivity to cold. Women often complain they "don't feel right." Since thyroid hormones regulate the way the heart beats and moves oxygen in the blood, inadequate amounts result in fatigue or having less stamina. The liver is less able to clear cholesterol from the blood when thyroid hormones are low, and the intestines slow down, causing constipation.

Growth of nails, skin, and hair is slowed, white patches may appear on your skin, you may lose hair from the outer edges of the eyebrows, and you may find your hair thinning. Because your muscles depend on thyroid, you may experience muscle stiffness, cramping, and weakness. Increased snoring occurs with some people.

As if all this wasn't enough, hypothyroidism may make you depressed, moody, forgetful, and unable to concentrate. Periods can become heavy or light, and you may retain fluid—all symptoms shared with menopause. Hypothyroidism must be treated to avoid long-term damage to the heart and kidneys and a deterioration of your general health. Fortunately, treatment is relatively simple, and proper medication dosage can usually be obtained within one to three months.

Careful regulation of one's dosage is important because excess thyroid replacement can interfere with calcium absorption and cause bone loss. For this reason, some women with hypothyroidism are advised to take ERT or HRT.

Thyroid bioavailability can be affected by malabsorptive states and also by interactions with other drugs, such as those that lower cholesterol and antacids containing aluminum hydroxide. Since true hypothyroidism cannot be reversed, daily medication must be taken for the rest of your life.[2]

Hyperthyroidism is less common than an underfunctioning thyroid gland. But this, too, can easily be mistaken for menopause. Nervousness and irritability, palpitations of the heart, hot flashes, fatigue, decreased menstrual flow, and sleep disturbances can convince the appropriate-aged female she is menopausal and needs estrogen. Three forms of therapy are available to treat hyperthyroidism: (1) radioactive iodine, (2) antithyroid drugs, and (3) surgery.

For the curious . . .
Signs of hypothyroidism:

sleepiness, fatigue   *depression*
loss of memory   *increase in weight*
unusually dry, coarse skin   *bloating, or puffiness*
goiter (enlarged thyroid)   *sensitivity to cold*
gradual personality change   *hair loss, sparseness of hair*

HYPOGLYCEMIA

Everyone has experienced the light-headedness, nausea, and general discomfort that comes with running out of fuel. People who suffer from hypoglycemia simply run out more frequently. A drop in blood sugar can cause you to shake, sweat, become anxious, feel dizzy, feel weak and tired, get a headache, have your heart pound, and get very irritable. True hypoglycemia is relieved within fifteen to twenty minutes by eating.

Unrecognized or uncontrolled hypoglycemia can resemble menopause, especially since it increases at midlife. Hypoglycemia often becomes worse as estrogen levels drop, making glycemic control more difficult. Eating smaller meals, avoiding alcohol, sugar, and high-glycemic carbohydrates, and ensuring adequate magnesium and chromium levels will help maintain blood sugar levels.

Sleeplessness, often caused by the hot flashes of menopause, can also be the result of a drop in blood sugar during the night. Eating a small bedtime snack containing a carbohydrate, protein, and fat can improve sleep by preventing a drop in blood sugar. For more details on how to maintain a steady blood sugar, see chapter 13.

293

BLAME IT ALL ON STRESS

There is hardly a menopausal symptom that can't be duplicated by stress manifesting itself in the body. Muscle and joint pain, bowel changes, insomnia, and fatigue can all be due to stress. Most important, stress modifies both the bioavailability and effectiveness of medications. Having been diagnosed with hypoglycemia and hypothyroidism, I can tell when stress levels are affecting my metabolism. My blood sugar level begins to do its own "dance," my thyroid begins to ache, and I am reminded to take stock of how I am handling all that is going on in my life. Reduction of stress, already discussed in chapter 15, is essential to maximize the effectiveness of any intervention you are using and to reduce symptoms in the first place.

IS MENOPAUSE JUST ONE BIG ATTACK OF PMS?

It is not uncommon for women to either experience PMS for the first time during the perimenopause, or to find their PMS pattern worsening. Whereas true PMS is limited to the second half of the cycle, perimenopausal symptoms occur during the entire cycle. The result is one big PMS month with symptoms that escalate toward the second half. It is not a pretty picture—and not fun to experience. If your PMS symptoms have increased or expanded to the whole month, you probably are perimenopausal.

A CLOSER LOOK AT "ADRENOPAUSE" AND GUT HEALTH

At A Woman's Place our approach to the journey of menopause changed radically when we realized the general health of our patients was just as significant in managing menopause as their changing hormone levels. Specifically, adrenal function and gut health were instrumental in the efficacy of any interventions. Our focus shifted from the menopause to functional medicine and moving our patients into optimal health. To borrow a phrase,

How Adrenal Hormones Are Interconnected

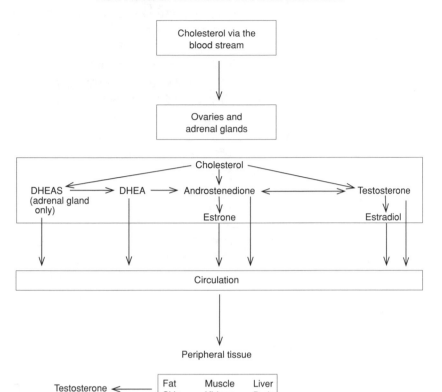

we wanted women to "be all they could be." Menopause itself merely provided timely motivation.

Throughout this text we have referred to the interconnectedness of all the body's hormones. We have alluded to the steroid hormones' ability to be "precursors" to other hormones. While the process is complex, and can be confusing, the above chart sheds light on sex steroid interconnectedness.[3]

Hormones to the Rescue

As we know by now, ovarian production of estrone, estradiol, and androgen are all reduced at menopause. Nevertheless, two androgens, androstenedione and testosterone, continue to be made. In fact they are produced more abundantly by the ovary than by the adrenal glands and are ultimately converted into most of a menopausal woman's estrogen. The other main androgens, DHEA and DHEAS, are produced primarily within the adrenals and are also reduced as we age. The drop in production by these four major androgens occurs at a slower rate than estrogen. However, the lowered androstenedione and testosterone levels are more closely tied to menopause than to aging.

The role of DHEA and DHEAS is not as clearly defined as those of androstenedione and testosterone, but they are believed to play an important function in maintaining health and vitality. Declining DHEA and DHEAS have been linked to lowered immune states and increased illness. Giving people DHEA is believed to have the ability to improve REM sleep, enhance memory, increase strength, and improve the sense of well-being. Consequently, adequate levels of DHEA may play a part in relieving common menopause complaints such as sleeplessness, regulating glycemic control and mood changes, and counteracting the estrogen loss by enhancing immunity.

Preventing Adrenopause

A woman who enters midlife with adrenal fatigue, often the result of chronic stress, illness, pain, or allergies, is likely to suffer more than the woman whose adrenals naturally compensate for the changing balance of androgens (and other precursor hormones that used to come from the ovaries). Her menopause is worsened by her "adrenopause." The important thing to remember is that failing ovarian function and decreased estrogen levels mean androgen precursors are more vital than ever. Their conversion to testosterone and estrogen (mainly estrone) occurs in the skin, fat tissue, muscles, kidneys, liver, and brain. Theoretically, maximizing their production could very well eliminate the need for estrogen replacement for some women, or at least dramatically reduce the intervention called for. *At midlife keeping adrenal glands healthy can ease the menopausal transition.*

The adrenal glands are attached above the kidneys. Besides the four main androgens, other hormones are also produced that

296

have a broad effect on the body. Stimulated by the pituitary hormones they balance sodium, potassium, and other minerals. Some affect the thyroid's ability to regulate our energy level. Still others modulate glucose, which is essential for good brain functioning and energy, amino acids, and fat metabolism. And then there is testosterone, associated with sexual responsiveness, libido, and a sense of well-being. A reduction in any of these hormones can seriously affect the quality of one's life and general state of wellness.

In times of stress the adrenals produce adrenaline and noradrenaline. These are the fight-or-flight hormones that give you "emergency" energy by supplying more oxygen, raising blood pressure, and increasing your heart rate. As blood levels of glucose and fatty acids rise, they cause your muscles to be flooded with extra nutrients. Unfortunately the fight-or-flight, or stress response, is a nondiscriminating responder. Any type of stress will prompt it into action.

Other emergency chemical alarms are also released when we are in pain; get angry or frustrated; have toxic exposure, allergies, or chronic infections; lack sleep; eat poorly; exercise too much; or are dealing with emotional strain, anxiety, or depression. Designed to react to emergencies, the end product of the stress response—cortisol—triggered by "nonemergencies," is left with nothing to do. Constant cortisol production increases the possibility of a number of chronic illnesses. After years of false alarms, the adrenals fatigue and function poorly or erratically. Eventually adrenal function is affected and what is known as "adrenal burnout" occurs. Improving adrenal health, therefore, is an indirect but vital way to enhance health in general and will specifically aid in adjustment to menopausal changes.

Too Many Stressors, Too Much Cortisol

Unrelenting production of cortisol brings women into the office with complaints of being unable to sleep, being hungry, having a series of infections (including yeast infections), and fatigue. Those most affected suffer from severe allergies, general aches and pains, and degenerative diseases like arthritis. They feel irritable, have problems with memory, suffer headaches, and are frequently unable to tolerate alcohol.

Such women are miserable, and menopause seems the likely culprit. In reality, menopause is only coincidental. Hormone replacement may bring some relief, but to their disappointment and frustration, does not "fix" them. Their distress is accentuated by the fact that medical tests, designed to measure disease states and not function, report that nothing is wrong. They are the "walking wounded," and there seems to be no explanation for it.

Dealing with Adrenal Problems

Adrenal function can be measured. One test, the Adrenal Stress Index, measures the fluctuations of salivary cortisol over a twenty-four-hour period under real life conditions.[4] A salivary DHEA(S) component measures the adrenal's capacity to produce androgens. This is important since, after extended chronic stress, cortisol output continues while androgen levels decrease. The plotted graphical results reveal if adrenal activity is normal, overfunctioning, or fatigued.

While exhausted adrenals have far-reaching health effects, treatment to revitalize and rebalance adrenal function is not at all radical. Depending on the degree of adrenal fatigue, supplementing with DHEA, pregnenolone, or cortisol may be required. Other aspects of treatment may include short-term use of phosphorylated serine derivatives. A high potency multivitamin is essential with additional B-complex, extra magnesium, and vitamin C. Botanical adaptogens, such as Siberian ginseng, can be used along with echinacea, silybum marianum, and licorice. Combinations of herbs balanced according to Chinese formularies are good choices because of Chinese medicine's tradition of focusing on adrenal and liver function for overall wellness.

The licorice used for healing is only vaguely related to those red and black sticks you nibble at the movies. The botanical licorice *(Glycyrrhiza glabra)* is a powerful adrenal stimulant. Combined with good health practices and reduction of stress, it can help prevent or reverse adrenal fatigue. By increasing the efficiency of the adrenal system, it stimulates production of adrenal hormones and increases the half-life of cortisol. As we've mentioned before, however, it should not be used all the time. Continued use can cause adrenal overstimulation, leading to Cushing's disease. Excess can cause bloating, weight gain, nervous anxiety, and heart palpitations. People with high blood pressure should not use licorice.

Mild exercise, stress management, and glycemic control are also part of recovery. Women with adrenal burnout will often complain of being excessively tired rather than refreshed by exercise. They must be very careful not to overdo aerobically. Stamina should be built by increasing walks, stretching, and the use of light weights. Prioritizing life so more time can be spent resting and in refreshing leisure activity speeds recovery. Finally, implementing a balanced and healthy diet that maintains glycemic control is the underpinning for renewed wellness. Note that most interventions for recovery from adrenopause are lifestyle changes and very much within your control. Given a chance and the right building materials, your adrenals will recover.

Yes, You've Got Guts, But . . .

Another overlooked source of fatigue, muscle and joint pain, digestive problems, food allergies, and general malaise is one's gastrointestinal and liver health. The primary role of your gastrointestinal tract is to break food down to a molecular level, absorb nutrients, and exclude toxins. It doesn't do its job very well when it is damaged. Malabsorption problems occur in which fat, protein, or carbohydrates (or all three) fail to enter the bloodstream efficiently through the intestine. Dysbiosis is the name given to the condition in which bowel flora is disordered and bacteria, yeasts, and/or protozoa alter nutrition and immune responses.

When problems exist with gut and liver function, your efforts at healthful eating and utilization of supplements and medications can become almost pointless. For example, when taken orally, estradiol converts to estrone within the gut wall. When it reaches the liver, its conversion continues and, ultimately, only a small proportion of what was originally ingested ends up circulating throughout the body within the bloodstream. If gut or liver function is poor, even less is available.

It is important that the bowel be able to "neutralize" toxins so they can be eliminated as soluble and safe by-products, preventing an overload of toxins in the liver. When the liver is overrun by persistent or potent toxins—from outside exposure or made within the body—the toxins accumulate. Essential fatty acids are expended, other metabolic changes result, and there is reduced energy production. Excess fatigue, food allergies or intolerances, autoimmune diseases like those affecting the thyroid, lowered immunity, and headaches are common outcomes of toxic buildup. The similarity of these symptoms to what many women experience at menopause can't be missed.

In general the body's inflammatory process is increased, escalating the odds of heart disease and, if the theories are right, Alzheimer's disease. Chronic illnesses, such as arthritis, are increasingly thought of as having a connection between digestive problems and the formation of immune responses and synovitis.[5] Other conditions suspected of having a "gut" connection include acne and eczema and chronic constipation or diarrhea.

Maintaining Balance in the Gut

A normal, functioning bowel contains somewhere between one hundred to four hundred different species of microscopic bacteria. Some of these varieties are beneficial and some are harmful. Maintaining good bowel flora involves making sure the "good bugs" outnumber the "bad." The small intestine, through which most of our food is absorbed, is lined with clinging bacteria—up to one hundred trillion of them.

Think, if you will, of the gut as a theater filled with thousands of seats. The patrons filling those seats are all legitimate ticket holders. What happens on the stage is what has been rehearsed and what the audience expects. In other words, the evening goes as planned. Intermission occurs and many of the ticket holders leave their assigned seats. In their absence, hooligans who have been hanging around the theater break in and take the vacated seats. When the patrons return, they find their reserved spaces occupied by persons who refuse to leave. Those who manage to oust the intruders may discover their seats have been damaged. The disruption affects the actors and dancers on stage, and the result is that the whole evening is less pleasant than it was planned to be.

This is essentially what happens in your gut. The legitimate ticket holders, the "good" bacteria, are in place until something comes along to dislodge them. That something could be antibiotics; corticosteroids; stress; poor diet; alcohol abuse; overuse of NSAIDS, aspirin, and other pain killers; illnesses; or toxic exposure. "Bad" bacteria, which are always present, don't overlook the opportunity to take the "good" seats, and something akin to chaos occurs. The new balance of bad-to-good bacteria can produce a variety of toxins, which among other effects, may contribute to widespread infections. Damage is done to the intestinal lining, allowing infections to occur within the lining itself, and the aftermath may manifest itself as disease far removed from the intestine.

For the curious . . . Symptoms that indicate you may have an imbalance of the bowel flora are changes in the stool and bowel patterns, intermittent abdominal pain, and feeling bloated. Antibiotics are the most common cause of bowel flora imbalance.

All My Tests Are Normal, but I Feel Awful

If assessment tests, your medical history, or an honest appraisal of your health suggest to you that intestinal and liver problems may be responsible for some of your unexplained aches and pains and general misery, there is help available. Minimally, you can reintroduce "good" bacteria into the bowel: lactobacillus species for the small intestine (acidophilus is most common, also bulgaricu, thermophilus) and bifidobacteria species for the large intestine (bifidus is most common, also longum, infantis, breve, etc.). We do not recommend, however, that you purchase these products off your grocer's shelf. Purified, isolated, live strains are available as capsules and powders from reputable health practitioners. They will have taken pre-

301

cautions to preserve them at the proper temperature, are observant of expiration dates, and only carry products with guarantees of adequate live counts. Acidophilus milk has the right idea but does not supply enough of the right strains of bacteria to do more than temporary good. Three trustworthy sources include:

> Metagenics: Ultra Flora Plus is a "one-stop" probiotic containing live bacteria and other factors to support their growth and activity.[6]
> InterPlexus, Inc.: HMF is a blend of viable complementary human species lactobacilli and bifidobacteria.[7]
> Ethical Nutrients: "Intestinal Care" and Intestinal Flora Factors

At A Woman's Place we recommend that patients use one of these products after a course of antibiotics, before surgery, after a time of severe stress, or anytime eating and lifestyle habits have been particularly erratic and unhealthful.

Working around Chemicals

Are you consistently exposed to pesticides and other chemicals known to be toxic? Is your health seriously compromised? Does your lifestyle include high stress and poor nutritional patterns? Do you simply not feel well for no apparent reason? If you answered yes to any of these questions, you may benefit from a more comprehensive approach to your gut and liver health. While fasting has typically been the method suggested for ridding the body of toxins, today there are safer, more tolerable, and more effective means.

At A Woman's Place we advise patients to follow a process developed by biochemist Jeffrey Bland, Ph.D.,

For the curious ... It is estimated that there are around one hundred thousand foreign chemicals (xenobiotics) to which we are exposed from drugs, pesticides, environmental pollutants, industrial chemicals, and food additives.

302

professor of chemistry at the University of Puget Sound, senior research scientist at the Linus Pauling Institute, and author of *The 20-Day Rejuvenation Diet Program*.[8] His program for restoring gut and liver function ameliorates their performance and reduces the toxic load in the body. Most important, it is backed by sound research. The plan is simple to follow and enables patients to carry out their everyday responsibilities with no disruption while producing outstanding results. There is one protocol directed toward liver functioning—UltraClear and UltraClear Plus—and one for improving gut health—Sustain. We have found, however, that improving the health of the digestive tract is sometimes enough to take the increased burden off the liver, allowing for its recovery and enhanced functioning without further intervention. Depending on assessment outcomes, patients are asked to use the powdered formulas mixed with water several times a day.[9] The UltraClear is the only patented formula to nutritionally modulate metabolic detoxification. UltraClear is unique in that it is merely giving the body what it needs to do its job of detoxification and gut healing, in contrast to the use of medications and herbal products that are most often prescribed and designed to modify normal function in the hope of bringing relief and healing.[10] Given the right support, the body heals itself.

Briefly, the concept is illustrated through The 4-R Gastrointestinal Support Plan,[11] which is designed to assist in the improvement or normalization of gut health and function, although its protocols apply for liver detoxification as well.

The 4R Gastrointestinal Support Plan

> Remove
> Replace
> Reinoculate
> Repair

1. *Remove:* If parasitic infection is suspected or shown to be present by laboratory tests, appropriate treatment is begun. Other pathogens, such as an overgrowth of yeast, are "removed" by natural or traditional medication. Laboratory testing aids in their

For the curious . . .
Probiotics are organisms or supportive substances that promote normal gastrointestinal function and health and inhibit the growth of undesirable bacteria. Fructooligosaccharides (FOS) is a fiberlike substance that feeds healthful bacteria. Other examples of probiotics are lactoferrin, which prevents harmful bacteria from getting the iron it needs, lactoperoxidase, which damages "bad" bacteria, and certain globulin proteins, which keep unhealthful bacteria from attaching to the intestinal wall.

proper identification. Many pathogens are normally in the bowel, but how many of them there are is as significant as what they happen to be. *Remove* also refers to elimination of foods to which an individual is allergic or sensitive, as well as food antigens that tend to stimulate inflammatory responses. Such a diet is called an oligoantigenic diet, commonly referred to as an elimination diet, which excludes dairy, citrus, red meats, pork, caffeine, alcohol, and foods containing gluten, among others.

2. *Replace:* Digestive factors, fiber, and/or enzymes are added to improve function and to boost the body's ability to properly break down food.

3. *Reinoculate:* With an oligoantigenic diet, enzyme factors, and other dietary supplements making a more favorable environment, reintroduction of "friendly" bacteria supported by probiotics helps reestablish a desirable balance of microflora.

4. *Repair:* Because damage has been done to the gut wall, substances known to aid in recovery of the gastrointestinal mucosa are included, and the individual is encouraged to eat foods with lots of nutrients and fiber such as cruciferous vegetables (broccoli, cauliflower, etc.) for their antioxidant effect.

The program lasts anywhere from two to six weeks, depending on individual response, and has proven to be life changing for a number of our chronically ill women. It results in greatly improved health for women less impaired. If nothing else, the elimination and reintroduction of foods to which many people are unaware of their sensitivities has proven eye-opening.

In our modern world, paying attention to the body's ability to handle pollutants is a necessary part of maintaining good health. While toxic exposure and the accompanying bowel disruption are often insidious health problems in comparison to the invasion and infection by bacteria, virus, or cancer, they nevertheless contribute to the slow but steady undermining of wellness. The relentless march toward poorer health, escalation of inflammatory processes, and degenerative diseases should not be ignored, although they usually are. This is why the focus of this book and our work at A Woman's Place has not been limited to relief of menopausal signs, symptoms, or angst.

A FOCUS ON FUNCTION

In conventional medicine, patients seek treatment from their physician when they are ill. The typical menopausal woman goes to her doctor when she is manifesting symptoms and probably feeling miserable. Her physician is trained to initiate care that relieves her symptoms and the focus is not on how her body is functioning. The doctor fixes only those problems verifiable on a laboratory test. But symptom relief and powerful interventions bring their own complications and do not necessarily translate into wellness. Early assessment, intervention, and treatment of diminished function, however, can forestall more serious health concerns, relieve symptoms, help a person feel better, jump-start the body into repairing itself, and move the individual toward her unique definition of optimal health.

Functional medicine, as such an approach is called, affects how genes ultimately express themselves, modifies biochemical pathways to support health, and focuses on restoring the body's function so the body can do what it was designed to do. Then the body can more effectively resist disease and eliminate toxins. It is more

305

likely to be a body that is full of energy and zest for living. With the addition of a balanced diet, good supplemental nutrition if needed, and lifestyle changes—as outlined in part 3 of this book—optimal living results. If these things are ignored, the reverse is apt to be true. Years of high-stress living, neglect and/or confusion over nutritional health, poor lifestyle habits, and toxic exposure result in increased vulnerability and less vitality.

If you are among the "walking wounded," suffer from chronic disease, or have long-standing health conditions or simply want to feel your very best, look first to your gut and liver health before increasing anti-inflammatories, antibiotics, or any other medications that relieve symptoms but mask *disease*. Find a health care partner who will look beyond symptoms and laboratory tests that measure when your condition has crossed the line to a categorically defined disease. Take one small step at a time, restore your health, and/or maximize your well-being by helping your body do what it was intended to do—keep itself well.

The traditional concept of health and disease suggests that we are well until we get sick. But the truth is that most of the time a slow decline in our well-being begins long before we decide we are sick and seek intervention. Along the way our health is impacted physically, emotionally, or spiritually by some occurrence. We appear to survive but underneath, all is literally not well. The process can be likened to a synome wave. It begins at a point far from the shore, the smooth surface belying the unseen turbulence underneath. The hidden churning hits the shore unexpectedly and causes unprepared for and unexpected chaos and destruction. For the body, this is when full-blown disease appears.

Research tells us that most Americans spend the last twelve years of their life fighting disease. Every one of us has better things to do. Menopause is the perfect time to take stock, review patterns, and begin interventions to ensure that the last third of life can be lived in a way that is of our own choosing.

Pearls of wisdom concerning menopause impostors . . .

1. A number of health problems can look like menopause or exacerbate menopausal symptoms.

2. Optimal health results from addressing the source of a problem rather than symptom relief.
3. Proper diagnosis is essential for maximum relief.
4. Correcting the way the body functions results in menopausal interventions working better and/or the need for them being reduced or eliminated.
5. Good gut and liver health makes a major contribution to overall health.

21

Reframing for the Future

When I'm counseling, I often ask the person I'm working with to "reframe" a situation over which they are distressed. For example, Linda was so distraught over the loss of a job she had held for twenty years that the tragedy of her situation overwhelmed her. Suggesting she reframe what had happened to her as "the best thing that could happen," initially made her laugh. Eventually, however, it led her to launch a new career that, while it had its rocky moments, brought her tremendous emotional satisfaction. Midlife brings losses but it also brings marvelous opportunities.

One great thing about aging is its power to force us to decide what is important. We have no choice but to reframe. Unlike other challenges we have faced, there is no backtracking, cash outlay, or creative thinking that can forestall getting older. Age is not to be denied but it no longer need be defined as infirm, over the hill, or the end of creative expression. Motivated to take stock of our health, to reduce responsibility and parenting, to no longer be ruled by fluctuations in hormones, the stage is set for new options.

Reframing does not ignore that many midlife women have obligations and responsibilities. But even that reality does not prevent the reevaluation of how one is living life. The internal and external pressures of having to keep doing what one has always done cries out to be examined and for the first time cannot be ignored.

TIME TO STOP RULING THE ROOST

For many women, taking an analytical look at their life means taking an honest look at the price one pays for "being in charge."

Something to think about . . .

Late Bloomers

Am I too fat?
Does my hair look right?
What dress should I wear?
Will I get a date to the prom?
Can I pass the test?
Has my essay enough research?
Why am I shaking about my report card?
Should I try out for the cheerleading team?
I am slim.
My hair has just been weaved.
The dress is the latest style.
I have a date to my favorite place tonight.
I just completed multiple budgets on time.
I'm confident about my Board presentation on
    Tuesday.
I got promoted last week.
I'm part of the corporate team.

Molly Seamons

What were you like as a teen?

In a very practical sense, whether a woman has worked in or out of the home, she has most likely "ruled her roost." Mom made the executive decisions that kept the family going on a day-by-day basis, counseled the children, looked after aging relatives, and was also the lover, friend, and confidant of her spouse. Her life has been lived as if everything within her universe depended on her. While she was heard to complain that the rest of the world wasn't doing their share, she nonetheless thrived and was motivated by the sense of urgency and importance her role demanded—even when she was the only one to acknowledge and appreciate it.

Maybe you are such a woman and at midlife you find yourself justifiably tired. Two truths become painfully evident—

(1) you can no longer manage living the way you always have and (2) you don't want to.

To continue "as always" feels burdensome in new ways and is neither satisfying nor necessary. Perhaps you have focused on a single goal so nothing else counted. Maybe you have met all the demands by mindlessly doing too many things at once. In either case, the penchant for getting it all done meant something had to be given up. That "something" was sleep, nutrition, taking care of health needs, and/or personal dreams and desires.

Most women tell themselves that those needs will be attended to after everything else is done. Then they'll rest, get a mammogram, take a vacation, go to school, or paint again. It may be new to think beyond being "ruler of her roost." It may be innovative to act beyond daily function and survival. But if contentment and optimal health are to be defining goals as one ages, women have no other choice.

The point is that midlife is a time when one is motivated to make changes. While there is little energy left for continuing life as usual, there is plenty that can be tapped into for new priorities. Since "ruler of her roost" is no longer the predominant role, the door is open to pursue other aspects of what a mature, wise woman has to offer. The resiliency and power that you have already demonstrated merely need to be creatively redirected. Creativity generates its own energy and is a far cry from a concept of slowing down or of the degeneration normally associated with aging.

FINDING A NEW SENSE OF BALANCE

But where do you begin? The good news is that small beginnings can lead to big changes. As a midlife woman you must first acknowledge that you have worked in some capacity for a very long time. But change is not confined to what you have done to fill your days. Every aspect of life must be examined. Such scrutiny includes the way you have approached your job, children, and relationships. Examination of your attitude toward your body and the kinds of things you have done or not done for your health are all a part of reframing.

Midlife is a time, first and foremost, for restoring balance. Depending on the way you have lived your life, balance is a very personal thing. Take one's job, for example. Women who enjoy their work have been found to be more open to change and are likely to feel better about life in general. These women may or may not include stopping work or changing jobs as options. Ironically, those who feel trapped or find little joy in their work have less confidence to change their situation. Unhappy women who are "stuck" are also likely to be heavier and less healthy.

If you have been guilty of "overcaring," you may need to work at putting yourself first for a change. If you have been caught up in the corporate world, you may find balance through service to others. Like many others, you may hunger for a reconnection with your spiritual roots and the traditions of your faith, this after years of rejection or avoidance of your religious life.

Whatever direction finding personal balance takes, it requires letting go of things that are no longer working or that are bogging you down. It is scary to examine the quality of relationships that are being maintained, the investment you're making in a job, and the commitment you have to a place or a lifestyle. But living optimally requires that you take a long, hard look at these things. Many of us have pursued goals and dreams based on conclusions reached in our youth and we have not reevaluated them since then. It is likely that some of the commitments you have made are no longer important. It is also possible that your energy is being drained by grudges, anger, and ill will.

For the first time, perhaps, choices must cease being automatic and become conscious. Activities that undermine your self-confidence, joy, personal growth, and health must be questioned. Asking, What is meaningful now? is an intelligent place to start. What do you really need to contribute? What practices and patterns will allow you to face aging with health and vigor? What ensures your being an active and fun grandparent? What restructuring is needed if a novel is to be written, serenity is to be experienced, world travel is to be enjoyed, school is to be attended, or golf is to be learned?

HOW CAN I TREAT MYSELF BETTER?

The bottom line is how can a woman treat herself better? More specifically, how can *you* treat *yourself* better? Coming up with a list isn't much of a challenge. Most women could use more rest, quiet times, less responsibility, and more attention paid to their health. Implementing such acknowledged necessities is far from simple, however. After a lifetime of overseeing others' well-being, and putting personal needs last, looking after yourself feels awkward. Yet it is essential.

Not only is increased care of yourself fitting, it is timely. Among all the other messages it sends us, menopause signals mortality. The sense that life as you know it is finite and that you are entering the third phase of your life span is a great motivator to make better use of the remaining time. The ill health or deaths of friends and family serve as painful reminders that each day must be made to count.

If you haven't learned it before, acknowledging your finite existence enables you to finally grasp what you have always known intellectually—that the present is all that can be counted on. Habits, thinking patterns, and activities that keep you focused either in the past or on the future need to be questioned.

Nelda reminisces about "her other life" as a modestly successful model and actress, while overlooking the need in her community for a drama club. The local high school has lost its funding for the arts and desperately needs experienced volunteers to establish an ongoing program. Nelda's inability to appreciate the present is a factor in her despair and her mournful feeling that life has passed her by. What keeps you from enjoying what you are doing while you are doing it or prevents you from trying new things?

TAKING TIME TO REFLECT

Midlife women must contemplate these and other questions. It's essential to begin by scheduling twenty to thirty minutes of unstructured time a day to think and evaluate one's situation. For many midlife women, finding even that small amount of time will be difficult and may result in guilt and anxiety. But space to think must be carved out. One must be quiet to hear the desire of the heart.

Additionally, there are methods more conducive to putting life in order than sitting numbed at your desk, sleeping, complaining to a friend, eating an extra treat, or spacing out in front of the television set. One of the most effective and pleasurable means for getting in touch with our feelings is to reconnect in some way with nature. If you are surrounded by plastic, add a real plant or fresh flowers to your room. Purchase a small fish tank for your desk. Enjoy a walk at lunch and take Rover for a hike. Visit a farmer's market or take a drive in the country. Sit in the park, go for a picnic, read a book on your patio—anything that awakens you to the vastness and beauty of nature.

How to Make Changes Happen

1. Take time
   a. Pencil in unstructured time on your calendar and consider it as sacred as any other appointment.
   b. Learn to appreciate silence. If quiet feels awkward, practice it in little doses. It may have been a long time since you have operated without background noise.
2. Reconnect with nature
   a. Rediscover walking in order to relate to the beauty and complexity of our world.
   b. Bring fresh flowers into the house—even one flower will do.
   c. Buy a goldfish.
3. Delegate work
   a. Ask others to do their share—unhook from the "ruler of the roost" syndrome.
   b. Eliminate tasks no one cares about but you.
4. Learn to say no
   a. Do only what you do best.
   b. Make choices based on what you value.
   c. Work with people you like and/or who energize you.
5. Gather information

    a. Consult others—there is strength in a multitude of counselors.

    b. Gather baselines from which health decisions affecting the quality of your life can be made.

6. Expect to grieve

    a. All changes are experienced as loss on some level, even healthy and desired ones. This is because something must be given up for something new to replace it.

    b. Grieving is a process involving denial, anger, bargaining, depression, and acceptance.

    c. Make peace with your life as you've lived it. There is no value in beating yourself up for past mistakes or regrets.

7. Make a timetable

    a. Small steps give encouragement and hope.

    b. Timetables imply a commitment while allowing for adjustments.

Simplifying and prioritizing your life is not nearly the mysterious process it first appears. Just below the surface is an awareness of parts of yourself that have heretofore not been allowed to be expressed. Once acknowledged, appropriate solutions will unfold naturally. Unfortunately this does not mean you can escape from having to be brutally honest and realistic. Real life means that there are real conflicts between what you may yearn to do and what you really value. Only you, for example, can decide if the long-held dream of studying painting in Paris is worth missing the birth of your first grandchild. Is "doing your thing" of greater value than a trip to Disneyland with all ages in tow, Thanksgiving dinner at your house, or last memories shared with aging parents? Only you will know.

In Search of a New Way to Live

Having gifted yourself with personal time and settings in which you are able to sincerely contemplate your situation, facilitate the process by continuing to unburden yourself. Ask for help with family chores and responsibilities you have handled without question or habitually executed as "ruler of the roost." If no one is willing to continue your legacy, consider letting those routines go. For instance, it may be nice to use Grandma's china at Thanksgiving, but if no one is willing to hand wash it, perhaps a new tradition is in order. This does not mean the things you do are not nice, convenient, and enjoyed—but they may not be valued. The fact that you are stressing yourself out over obligations in which you alone have a vested interest is a signal that those tasks need to be dropped.

Life really does go on, even when work, intensive traditions, or habits are eliminated or modified. But this is a lesson learned much too late for most women. Habits are hard to break. Routines will change only because a concerted effort is made to change them. It is also a struggle to break the habit of saying yes to worthy and good projects. But, for the first time, direction has to be defined not by the desires and demands of others, but by what you deem right for yourself.

What do you value? What do you do well? By midlife you already know. Don't struggle to be the treasurer of the local PTA when your strength is hospitality and meeting people. Don't agree to be in charge of the Sunday school at your church when your passion is to establish a garden for the homeless. People-pleasing decisions make no sense and result in unnecessary anxiety. Taking on extra projects at work or continually doing more than your share may be something you have come to expect of yourself, but does it have significance beyond being a workaholic? There is no end to the good and noble things you can do. But if you measure them by what is meaningful to you and by your strengths, you'll know immediately if they will eventually become burdens.

I'M LATE, I'M LATE FOR A VERY IMPORTANT DATE

Menopause is merciless in forcing a reappraisal of "Why the hurry?" The inability to maintain a breakneck pace is often what brings women to our clinic. Their goal is to repair whatever is causing their waning energy and diminished enthusiasm. That way, they assume they'll be able to return to life "as usual." Rather

315

than asking, "How can I treat myself better?" they are request-ing instead, "Fix me so I can keep up the rapid pace at which I've always lived my life." Our task is to help them see that their inabil-ity to live life as usual is a wake-up call for reevaluation.

"A TIME TO MOURN AND A TIME TO DANCE"

The sense of not having lived up to one's potential can have a number of origins. An overly demanding parent or belief in a harshly judgmental God may be setting the standard. These can be background thoughts, even though a woman is protesting, with seemingly good reason, that there is too much to do. Busy-ness is indeed a product of modern society and "timesaving" devices. If you stay too busy most of the time, however, you should question your motivation. Maintaining a sane and work-able schedule is rarely a problem when you are convinced and confident that you are doing what you should be doing. After all, don't you somehow find time for the things that matter to you?

Finally, appreciate the fact that change does not occur with-out grieving, because the familiar must be given up. There is loss even when there is wholehearted enthusiasm for living life dif-ferently. However, on the positive side, there is personal power expressed in deciding that things will be different.

Mourning is a necessary part of letting go and moving on. Grieving is a country road that seems to meander interminably before one's destination is reached. Much has been written about the stages of grieving, and it is recommended that you familiar-ize yourself with the steps of denial, anger, bargaining, depres-sion, and acceptance that accompany it.

But, you protest, "My menopause is a time of vibrancy and rejuvenation." The fact that losses must be mourned does not deny the new opportunities that are simultaneously presenting themselves. Remember, that is what reframing is all about. The reality, however, is that even with a great attitude and exciting possibilities, changes are necessary. At midlife, we are faced with different demands on our time, a diminished value in the mar-

316

ketplace, our children's emancipation, coming to terms with what did or didn't get accomplished in our lives, and the illness and death of family members and friends. We may also be struggling with a disappointing marriage, the loss of fertility without children, disappointment of not having lived the noble life we planned, violation of personal moral standards, energy wasted in mean-spirited, jealous, or evil thoughts, and changing physical performance.

What would you add to the list?

WHY WAS I PLACED ON THIS PLANET?

Many women may have on their list changes in their physical attractiveness.

Complaints of extra pounds and new wrinkles are common. But there is a positive side. Now the focus of determining worth can shift to a study of the total person. Whereas men have always accepted that they are more than the image they see in the mirror, women are finally compelled to see themselves in their totality. For certain, it is a time to let go of competition with other women. Value lies in being loved and accepted, not because societal standards of beauty are met, but because the midlife woman is interesting—she has lifetime achievements, depth of character, and absorbing experiences. Shifting the standard for acceptability enables self-worth to be based on a much deeper and significant concept. The question of why you are on this planet is the significant one. Detours and distractions that keep you focused on yourself or mired in the everyday no longer need be stumbling blocks to understanding spirituality or finding a true criterion of worth.

DISCOVERING SPIRITUALITY

Grasping the significance of the spiritual basis for life is the reason the last third of your lifetime holds the potential to be richer and more fulfilling than any other. The call to live beyond the immediate is a roar for some, and a still, small, but unrelenting voice for others. At midlife, the seed for spiritual growth has been planted and the time has come to water it.

317

Balance is a source of creativity and energy, which motivates you to attend to all aspects of your life. A lifetime of having focused on the externals has proven full of shortcomings, especially in contrast to a rich inner life. By denying age, we imply that something is wrong with growing more experienced, accepting, spiritual, knowledgeable, wise, simple, and worldly at the same time. Growing older and wiser helps us to learn that, in comparison to the big picture, what we have achieved that affects either the world at large or our own smaller world is increasingly insignificant.

REFRAMING HEALTH

Reframing is not confined to your emotional, psychological, and spiritual life. Taking a new look at how you have viewed your body and approached your health care is also in order. The goal is not to hang on to youth. Staying perpetually young is not growing old gracefully, neither is extending our ability to reproduce. The capacity to have children is not the only thing that makes a woman valuable to society, and we must not act as if it is. Our midlife challenge is to maintain health and to live productively, while letting go of one phase of life and embracing a new one.

Maintaining health while transitioning to a new, fruitful, and generative stage of life brings up many questions and concerns. *The Menopause Manager* offers the assurance that menopausal complaints are common and will go away with time. Not all women find them problematic, but enough do for difficulties to be addressed realistically and compassionately. We have also attempted to clarify why symptoms occur and how certain interventions alleviate them. An emphasis has been placed on distinguishing the difference between the signs of menopause and other health concerns that tend to manifest at midlife, so that interventions will be appropriate and as effective as possible.

The need for a health care partner should be very clear. What you are to do is no longer solely in the hands of a physician. This is true for a variety of reasons. With new information as close as the Internet, a physician is no longer perceived as someone who holds all the cards in the game of your life, especially since he or she increasingly must practice under the constraints of a rapidly changing health care system. Along with the right and necessity to be an active partner in health comes responsibility on your part. You must be an educated consumer. And if your physician no longer has the final word on your health care, make sure the local health food store clerk or the five o'clock news doesn't either.

The advice you need may come from a family doctor or from a multitude of health care providers. But whoever they are, you need them to be flexible and supportive partners in choosing a variety of solutions. Base your decisions on risk factors, family history, perceived personal risk, willingness to be consistent with any plan you decide on, well-established research, finances, and your personal values.

Knowledge is the key to good decisions, and the chance for good health is increased when information has been gleaned from a variety of sources. There are no guarantees, however. Good decisions with poor outcomes are possible. Hopefully *The Menopause Manager* has shown you that menopausal intervention, if needed to make life more bearable, as protection from inherited health risks, or taken as prevention, really does make a positive difference. Women who have completed menopause already remind us that the menopause journey does end and the destination isn't a disappointment. Perhaps one of the midlife icons, French actress Brigitte Bardot said it best, "It's sad to grow old, but nice to ripen."

APPENDIX A

Questions and Answers

Q: DOES MENOPAUSE MEAN MY OVARIES NO LONGER WORK?

A: Walnut-sized ovaries are the glands involved both in puberty and menopause. At puberty, ovarian production of the hormones estrogen and progesterone sets in motion the rhythmic pattern that results in the monthly maturation of an egg from a follicle in the ovary. Menopause occurs when there are no eggs left to be released and hormone production is diminished.

Your ovaries, however, continue to function. The outer part of the ovary, the theca, is where the eggs grow and is what regresses at midlife. The inner stroma remains active and is the site of continued hormone production, particularly, androstene-dione, which can be converted to estrone, testosterone, and dehy-droepiandrosterone (DHEA), which can convert to testosterone, progesterone, and estradiol.

Q: WHAT HAPPENS TO ALL THOSE EGGS?

A: One would think that eggs would never be in short supply considering that soon after conception, a baby girl's ovaries contain one to two million of them. Yet by menopause there are none left. Throughout a woman's lifetime three hundred to four hundred eggs mature and are released. Obviously, only a few are fertilized and fewer still result in the birth of a baby. What happens to all the other eggs? A variety of things: Most are reabsorbed; some are destroyed by toxins like nicotine; others simply fail to mature.

Q: HOW DO THE OVARIES KNOW WHAT TO DO?

A: The ovaries are part of the endocrine gland system, and the hormones they release go directly into the bloodstream. Chemical messengers called neurotransmitters under the direction of

320

the brain control their function. Specifically, the hypothalamus, located at the base of the brain, receives and directs input and sends orders out, responding to stimuli from within and without the body. Its production of gonadotropin releasing hormone is directed to the pituitary, a pea-sized gland directly under the hypothalamus. The pituitary releases two gonadotropins called follicle-stimulating hormone (FSH) and luteinizing hormone (LH). The egg follicle ripens under the influence of FSH and the egg matures and is released as a result of LH. No one knows why one egg is chosen over another. The buildup of estrogen and progesterone that occurs as the follicle matures and the egg is released stimulates neurotransmitters to produce endorphins that feed back to the hypothalamus, which in turn stimulates the pituitary to release or stop LH and FSH production.

Q: HOW DOES THE OVARY PRODUCE ESTROGEN AND PROGESTERONE?

A: The cells that surround the follicle and ovum produce estrogen. They also cause multiplication of cells and the buildup of the uterine lining during the first half of the cycle. The increased level of estrogen makes its way back to the hypothalamus, which again orders the pituitary to release another jolt of FSH and a bigger dose of LH. The LH causes the follicle to release the ripened egg. The empty follicle is called the corpus luteum and produces both estrogen and progesterone.

The rising level of progesterone essentially manages the second half of the cycle, maturing the lining of the uterus while modifying the estrogen effect. Progesterone does this by slowing down the multiplication of cells in the uterine lining. This is a relevant point to remember in terms of menopause and consideration of hormone replacement. It is estrogen that prompts multiplication of cells in the uterus and progesterone that prevents overgrowth.

After the release of the egg, rising progesterone levels signal the brain, via the hypothalamus and pituitary, to stop the ovary from producing estrogen by decreasing FSH production. Without fertilization, LH decreases, the corpus luteum dissolves, estro-

321

gen and progesterone levels drop, the lining of the uterus sheds, and a menstrual period begins. Declining estrogen and progesterone signals the need for production of FSH and the cycle repeats itself.

Q: What causes signs of menopause?

A: As a woman enters the perimenopause, fewer follicles exist and the process of maturation of the egg becomes somewhat erratic. Some periods are unchanged while others are lighter, heavier, longer, shorter, or in some other way different from what is typical for that individual. Fluctuating and lessening levels of estrogen and progesterone explain these and other changes.

When hormone levels are low, the pituitary increases the level of FSH and LH trying to force a follicle to mature, release an egg, and carry on as usual. Without enough progesterone the uterine lining continues to grow until it outstrips its blood supply and sheds erratically, causing the woman to experience sporadic and occasionally heavy bleeding. Low levels of both hormones may result in the same woman having light but persistent spotting throughout the next month. High estrogen levels are known to make a woman feel anxious; high progesterone levels result in depression. Low levels of both contribute to mood swings, irritability, and loss of a sense of control and well-being.

Q: How do you know menopause is really happening?

A: When hormone levels drop to the point that the lining of the uterus does not grow, periods stop altogether. One way a doctor determines if a woman is menopausal is to measure the FSH level in the blood. Elevated levels mean the pituitary is working hard to stimulate follicles that are too damaged to respond fully or simply no longer in existence. When all egg follicles are depleted, a woman is postmenopausal.

Measuring the precise levels of estrogen, progesterone, testosterone, and DHEA can be done. Such tests must be repeated at different times in the cycle to be accurate and because of the expense are not always recommended.

Tests that prove a woman is menopausal:

1. *Endometrial biopsy.* The lining shows anovulation effects and is thin and flat.
2. *Sonogram.* Measurement of the thickness of the uterine lining reveals if there are endometrial changes due to follicular activity.
3. *Measurement of the follicle-stimulating hormone.* A result of 40+ indicates menopause. Symptoms can occur from 20+. In many women FSH levels rise well before periods cease. The rise is picked up most frequently during the first half of the cycle and may not show up during the second half.
4. *Measurement of the luteinizing hormone.* From one to three years after FSH levels rise, LH is elevated.
5. *Saliva and blood tests.* These measure individual hormone levels.

Q: DOES WEIGHT AFFECT HOW YOU EXPERIENCE MENOPAUSE?

A: Androstenedione and testosterone, stored in the fat of a woman's body, can be converted into estrogen. Obviously, a very heavy woman may produce considerable estrogen, enough to put her at higher risk for breast and uterine cancer. Her thinner sister may experience more menopausal symptoms because her body cannot compensate for the loss of ovarian estrogen since she has fewer fat cells through which estrogen can be made. The lesson to be learned is to neither be too thin or too heavy at midlife. A modest weight gain at menopause might be naturally programmed into being a woman.

Q: MY DOCTOR NEVER MENTIONED THE "PERIMENOPAUSE." DOES IT REALLY EXIST?

A: There are few things more frustrating than finding one's reality challenged. A physician's refusal to consider menopause as a source of medical concerns is a justifiable complaint that we have heard at our menopause clinic over and over again. The classic line of dismissal is, "If you are younger than fifty and your periods haven't stopped for a year, you can't be menopausal." The truth is, the perimenopausal journey can begin surprisingly and subtly early, with first changes largely undetected by the woman and certainly not connecting in her mind with menopause. Yet the perimenopause simply doesn't exist for many physicians or is not seen as a time when intervention is called for.

Women rarely seek professional help unless their symptoms are worsening to the point that their quality of life is affected or because their family history warrants it. Consequently the physical upheaval and the emotional strain of not knowing what is happening to a body a woman has been an expert on for a lifetime forces her to conclude any number of things. The perimenopausal woman may decide she is going crazy and may fear that she will never feel good or be in control again. She may obsess over some as yet undiagnosed but imagined disease. In the end, she may dismiss the medical community as a source of healing and comfort. It should be a cause of concern to physicians that many women put more trust in the seventeen-year-old clerk at the health food store than in their years of medical training, or could it be the clerk listens more carefully?

Q: WHAT CAUSES MENOPAUSE IN THE PRIME OF LIFE?

A: As yet, no one knows exactly why a relatively young woman enters menopause prematurely. It is estimated that one woman out of one hundred will enter menopause before forty.[1] There is evidence of a genetic connection in some families. There are suspicions of autoimmune disorders as the cause, especially since they increase at midlife. Perhaps the body produces some not yet understood antiovarian antibodies. Poor diets and stress have been implicated because of their contribution to allergic responses and systemic yeast problems.

There is no debate about one cause of premature menopause, and that is smoking. Smoking inhibits liver function by blocking liver enzymes needed for estrogen production and by chemically damaging eggs. If you have smoked in the past but stopped, the negative effects may be modified, compared to what they would be if you were still smoking.

Q: WHAT HAPPENS WHEN MENOPAUSE IS DUE TO SURGERY?

A: For obvious reasons, women who undergo surgical menopause generally experience severe symptoms. The suddenness of dramatically reduced hormone levels leaves the body no time to accommodate. Removal of the tubes and ovaries (bilateral sal-pingo-oophorectomy) creates the most havoc, but other procedures are now known to also have an effect. A hysterectomy in which the tubes and ovaries are left in place will trigger menopause in 30 percent of women within two years. Dr. Philip Sarrel, in a 1996 article in *The OB/GYN Journal,* reported that 25 percent of such women, on objective endocrine measures, will become menopausal within three months and 50–60 percent within three years of surgery, no matter what their age. The potential impact of surgery on the system is evident, when occasionally after a tubal ligation for birth control, a hormonal adjustment time is needed because of the altered blood flow to the ovary, although most women find their bodies eventually adjust.

Women who must undergo chemotherapy for cancer find menopause hastened because the therapy works on cells most likely to divide and grow and it thus targets the eggs in the ovaries. Radiation of the pelvis destroys follicles and can cause vaginal scarring, making the area fibrous and tough, thereby preventing the walls from stretching as before or it can result in a thin and fragile vaginal lining. Besides the struggle to survive cancer, the woman must instantaneously adjust to menopause.

Q: THE ADS SAY TAKE TUMS AS A CALCIUM SUPPLEMENT BUT MY OB/GYN SAYS NO WAY. WHOM DO I BELIEVE?

A: There is considerable controversy about the absorbability of various calcium supplements. The dispute begins with how readily a calcium supplement breaks down. Most calcium is in the form of an insoluble salt, which depends on hydrochloric acid from the stomach to alter it so it can be absorbed in the small intestine.

While the makers of Tums tout its absorbability, the medication is designed to reduce stomach acid (hydrochloric acid)—the ingredient necessary to make calcium soluble. Since we tend to have less stomach acid as we age, for older women the argument for the importance of the preliminary step of calcium breakdown has credence. There is no question that antacids that contain aluminum inhibit absorption of phosphorus and increase excretion of calcium.

As a group, nutritionists are pretty united concerning the importance of high solubility for any calcium supplement you take, while other health practitioners question its importance.[2] The actual absorption of calcium into the bloodstream occurs through the small intestine, which is not acidic. That may be considered proof that acid is not essential for calcium breakdown or it may emphasize the importance of early breakdown before it reaches the small intestine. The objection to Tums is also that it lacks magnesium and other trace minerals, necessary for calcium absorption and bioavailability.

Q: I READ THE PACKAGE INSERT AFTER MY DOCTOR PRESCRIBED HORMONES AND I NEVER FILLED MY PRESCRIPTION.

A: The list of catastrophes that may occur as a result of taking a medication are there because the law requires that any and everything that could remotely happen be disclosed. Remember, however, if you drink enough, you can overdose on water. To keep your perspective when reading the list, make note of the percentage of occurrence. While participating in a trial for FDA approval, if a drug was ever associated with someone's toenail curling, it must be listed as a potential effect even if further exploration was not done to note if the "toenail curler" also overdosed on garlic while taking the medication.

Most important, what is on the list is what was known at the time the product was approved by the FDA. Drug companies rarely change the labeling as new information accumulates because redoing the FDA process would be like volunteering to go over your last ten years of taxes with the IRS. You may have nothing to hide but the process is overwhelming. For many classes of drugs, inserts are basically the same. What is reflected in a multiple products class insert is designed so as not to give any one company a product advantage.

Many of the most vocal opponents to hormone replacement use these inserts as proof positive of the detrimental effects of hormones. If you are looking for scientific backing to make an informed decision, product inserts are not your best source. For example, reliable and new research exists that has shown estrogen to be protective against heart disease, and it is the major reason hormone replacement is recommended, and yet opponents quote "from the drug company's own research," asserting that hormone replacement causes heart disease, high blood pressure, and a myriad of other problems.

A sample warning on estrogen replacement inserts cautions people about taking ERT if they have breast cancer, fibrocystic breast disease, cancer of the uterus, abnormal blood clotting, or any heart disease, high blood pressure, kidney disease, asthma, skin allergy, epilepsy, migraine headache, diabetes, depression, gall bladder disease, and fibroids. A study done through the American College of Obstetrics and Gynecology (ACOG) bulletin on contraindications for HRT found 50 percent of women at least some time in their history had some reason not to take HRT, based on this expanded list.[3]

Q: DR. SUSAN LOVE IS AN EXPERT ON BREAST CANCER. SHE THINKS THAT IN MOST CASES WOMEN DO NOT NEED AND SHOULD NOT USE HORMONES. WHAT AM I SUPPOSED TO BELIEVE?

A: As former director of the Revlon–U.C.L.A. Breast Cancer program and an advisor to the National Institutes of Health's Women's Health Initiative, Susan Love, M.D., is an authority on breast cancer in women. She is correct when she calls for women to take greater initiative in good health practices and lifestyle changes. No one will argue that exercising and eating more soy can be beneficial. But in evaluating what Dr. Love has to say, balance is the issue. When speaking of hormone replacement, she tends to overstate the risks and understate the benefits. She quickly dismisses the solid evidence of the protective effect of HRT for cardiovascular and osteoporotic problems by stating that the benefits have been observed in white middle class women, who get better medical care anyway. She ignores reanalysis that addresses such bias while selectively overlooking the bias implied in her conclusion that soy, not hormones, is what is needed since Japanese women have less breast cancer. She does not consider genetic homogeneity and other lifestyle differences when drawing this conclusion.

Dr. Love also overstates the effect of estrogen on breast cancer. Using the fact that conditions that reduce a woman's lifetime exposure to estrogen, such as having lots of children and beginning periods late, reduce the breast cancer risk, she deduces that estrogen equals breast cancer. But the greatest incidence of breast cancer occurs when estrogen production is reduced after menopause. Such is the complexity of its etiology. As discussed in chapter 19, research is unclear on the link between estrogen and breast cancer. If anything, there is a small increase of breast cancer after long-term use. Statistically, only those with the highest risk of breast cancer and no heart disease risk have nothing to gain and perhaps a negative effect on their health by taking hormones. While Dr. Love says "there are actually three times as many deaths from breast cancer as there are from heart disease" in women under seventy-five, this is simply not true, and she has failed to address this fact when confronted with it. The truth is that between the ages of forty-five and fifty-four the death rate due to heart disease is 1.4 times that of breast cancer. Between the ages of fifty-five and sixty-four, the death rate due to heart disease is 3 times that of breast cancer; between sixty-five and seventy-four it's 5.5 times greater, and over age seventy-five, it's 20 times greater (M. Gladwell, "The Estrogen Question: How Wrong Is Dr. Susan Love?" *The New Yorker* [June 9, 1997], 54–61). Her statistics are reversed. In women under seventy-five there are 3 times more deaths from heart disease than from breast cancer. At every age more women die from heart disease than from breast cancer.

Indeed, not all women need or should take hormones, but the decision should be an informed one, based on knowledge of personal risk factors, lifestyle choices, and family history, including the most recent risk factors linked with estrogen, such as Alzheimer's disease and colon cancer.

Vitamin and Mineral Intake

Recommended Vitamin Intake

Vitamin	Range for Adults
Vitamin A (retinol)	5,000 IU
Vitamin A (from beta-carotene)	5,000–25,000 IU
Vitamin D	100–400 IU
Vitamin E (d-alpha tocopherol)	100–800 IU
Vitamin K (phytonadione)	60–300 mcg.
Vitamin C (ascorbic acid)	100–1,000 mg.
Vitamin B_1 (thiamin)	10–100 mg.
Vitamin B_2 (riboflavin)	10–50 mg.
Niacin	10–100 mg.
Niacinamide	10–30 mg.
Vitamin B_6 (pyridoxine)	25–100 mg.
Biotin	100–300 mcg.
Pantothenic acid	25–100 mg.
Folic acid	400 mcg.
Vitamin B_{12}	400 mcg.
Choline	10–100 mg.
Inositol	10–100 mg.

Recommended Mineral Intake

Mineral	Range for Adults
Boron	1–6 mg.
Calcium	250–1,250 mg.
Chromium	200–400 mcg.
Copper	1–2 mg.
Iodine	50–150 mcg.
Iron[*]	15–30 mg.
Magnesium	250–500 mg.
Manganese	10–15 mg.
Molybdenum	10–25 mcg.
Potassium	200–500 mg.
Selenium	100–200 mcg.
Silica	1–25 mg.
Vanadium	50–100 mcg.
Zinc	15–45 mg.

[*] Men and postmenopausal women rarely need supplemental iron.

Charts are adapted from *Encyclopedia of Nutritional Supplements,* copyright © 1996 by Michael Murray, Rocklin, Calif.: Prima Publishing. Buy or order at better bookstores or call 800-632-8676.

www.primapublishing.com

Appendix C

Questions to Ask about Botanicals

The best way to know what you are getting when you use herbs is to know the company that packages them. To ensure your botanicals (herb-based supplements) are pure and properly prepared, ask the following questions.

1. Is the company well established with a good reputation?
2. Are there trained herbologists and/or researchers in nutrition and medicine on staff?
3. Are there M.D.s or Ph.D.s in the company?
4. Does the company have an operating plan that includes on-site inspections and visits to its suppliers or vendors?
5. Are there clear, published quality control guidelines?
6. Do raw materials have a certificate of analysis?
7. Are materials and/or finished products tested on a regular basis according to specified guidelines?
8. Does testing measure for heavy metals, bacteria, and degradation of herbal materials?
9. Are products tested for concentrations of active compounds when guidelines exist?
10. Are formulas based on established protocols and/or scientific data?
11. Are the instructions for use clear?
12. Is packaging appropriate to protect quality?
13. Does the label specify the portion of the plant from which the herb was taken?
14. Are genus and species name included?
15. Is there an expiration date?
16. Does the company have educational material available as well as information on its specific formulations?

Notes

INTRODUCTION: *SEEING THE BIG PICTURE*

1. Mark Percival, D.C., N.D., is an inspiration to anyone who seeks wellness and/or wants to help others reach their level of optimal health. He has had a great influence on A Woman's Place. Health Coach Systems International is located at 3 Waterloo St., New Hamburg, Ontario, Canada NOB 2G0, 519-662-2520.

2. *1988 Surgeon General's Report on Nutrition and Health.*

CHAPTER 1: *WHAT OTHERS HAVE DONE*

1. Dr. Tori Hudson, a leading naturopathic physician, is a professor at the National College of Naturopathic Medicine, Portland, Oregon. She is author of *Gynecology and Naturopathic Medicine: A Treatment Manual,* 3d ed. (Aloha, Oreg.: TK Publications, 1994).

CHAPTER 3: *BLEEDING IRREGULARITIES*

1. P. Roma, "A Simple Strategy for Managing Perimenopausal Bleeding," *Contemporary OB/GYN* 42, no. 5: 161–62.

2. E. Goldman, "Transvaginal US First Choice for Abnormal Bleeding," *OB.GYN. News* 31, no. 10 (May 15, 1996): 1–2.

3. P. Peck, "Endometrial Stripe Alone No Basis for Biopsy," *OB.GYN. News* 25 (1996): 25.

CHAPTER 4: *HOT FLASHES*

1. H. Adlercreutz, T. Fotsis, C. Bannwart et al., "Determination of Urinary Lignans and Phytoestrogen Metabolites, Potential Antiestrogens and Anticarcinogens in Urine of Women on Various Habitual Diets," *Steroid Biochemistry* 25 (1986): 791–97.

2. Schaper and Brummer, "Remifemin: A Plant-based Gynecological Agent." A copy of the article may be obtained from GmbH and Co., KG, P.O. Box 6111, 60/38251 Salzgitter, Germany; Tel. 0 53 41/307 800; FAX 0 53 41/307-413.

3. T. Tamkin, "Royal Jelly Can Trigger Severe Allergic Reaction," *Medical Tribune Clinical Rounds* (March 7, 1996): 9.

4. Y. Wyon, R. Lindgren, T. Lundeberg, and M. Hammar, "Effects of Acupuncture on Climacteric Vasomotor Symptoms, Quality of Life, and Urinary Excretion of Neuropeptides among Postmenopausal Women," *Menopause* 2, no. 1 (1995): 3–12.

5. C. L. Loprinzi, J. C. Michalak, R. N. Quella et al., "Megestrol Acetate for the Prevention of Hot Flashes," *New England Journal of Medicine* 331 (1994): 346–52.

CHAPTER 5: *VULVA, VAGINA, AND UTERUS CHANGES*

1. M. Messina and S. Barnes, "The Roles of Soy Products in Reducing Risk of Cancer," *Journal of the National Cancer Institute* 83 (1991): 541–46.

2. "Yogurt Ingestion Prevents Recurrent Vaginitis and BV," *The Female Patient* 22 (February 1997): 40.

3. W. Stoll, "Phytopharmacon Influences Atrophic Vaginal Epithelium: Double-blind Study Cimicifuga vs. Estrogenic Substances," *Therapeuticum* 1 (1987): 23–31.

CHAPTER 6: *BLADDER AND URETHRAL CHANGES*

1. E. Versi, L. Cardozo, J. Studd et al., "Urinary Disorders and Menopause," *Menopause* 2, no. 2 (1995): 94.

2. M. Limouzin-Lamothe, H. Mairon, C. R. B. Joyce et al., "Quality of Life after Menopause: Influence of Hormone Replacement Therapy," *American Journal of Obstetrics and Gynecology* 170 (1994): 618–24.

3. K. E. Nilsson and G. M. Heimer, "Ultra-low-dose Transdermal Estrogen Therapy," *Menopause* 1, no. 4 (1994): 191–97.

CHAPTER 8: *FATIGUE AND SLEEPLESSNESS*

1. J. Blanc, E. Barrager, R. Reedy, and K. Bland, "A Medical Food-Supplemented Detoxification Program in the Management of Chronic Health Problems," *Alternative Therapies* 1, no. 5 (November 1995): 18.

2. A. J. Block, P. G. Boysen, J. W. Wynne et al., "Sleep Disordered Breathing and Nocturnal Oxygen Desaturation in Postmenopausal Women," *American Journal of Medicine* (1980): 69–75.

3. "Menopause Disrupts Sleep Function," *OB.GYN. News* (January 1, 1996): 10.

CHAPTER 9: *MEMORY, MOOD SWINGS, AND DEPRESSION*

1. E. Barrett-Conner and D. Kritz-Silverstein, "Estrogen Replacement Therapy and Cognitive Function in Older Women," *Journal of the American Medical Association* 269 (1993): 2637–41.

2. B. Sherwin, "Hormones, Mood, and Cognitive Functioning," *Obstetrics and Gynecology* 87, no. 2, suppl. (February 1996): 20s–26s.

3. B. Sherwin, "Memory in Postmenopausal Women: What Is the Role of Estrogen?" *Menopause Management* (1993): 16–18.

4. B. Gates, "ERT Boosts Mental Performance, Brain Activity," *OB.GYN. News* 31, no. 11 (1996): 16.

5. M. Tucker, "Equilin May Help Older Women Preserve Memories," *OB.GYN. News* 31, no. 11 (June 1, 1996): 16.

6. J. C. Montgomery, L. Appleby, M. Brincat et al., "Effects of Oestrogen and Testosterone Implants on Psychological Disorders in the Climacteric," *Lancet* i (1987) 297–99.

7. P. Schmidt and D. Rubinow, "Menopause-related Affective Disorders: A Justification for Further Study," *American Journal of Psychiatry* 148 (1991): 844–52.

B. Sherwin and M. Gelfand, "Sex Steroids and Affect in the Surgical Menopause: A Double-blind, Cross-over Study," *Psychoneuroendocrinology* 10 (1985): 325–35.

8. G. T. Bungay, M. P. Vessey, and C. K. McPherson, "Study of Symptoms in Middle Life with Special Reference to the Menopause," *British Medical Journal* ii (1980): 181–83.

9. A. L. Dunn and R. K. Dishman, "Exercise and Neurobiology of Depression," *Exercise Sport Science Review* 19 (1991): 41.

10. B. Maoz et al., "HRT and Psychological Distress," *Menopause* 1, no. 3 (1994): 137–41.

11. L. A. Palinkas and E. Barrett-Conner, "Estrogen Use and Depressive Symptoms in Postmenopausal Women," *Obstetrics and Gynecology* 80 (1992): 330–36.

CHAPTER 10: *SEX AND HEADACHES*

1. W. H. Utian and I. Schiff, "NAMS-Gallup Survey," *Menopause* 1, no. 1 (1994): 39–48.

2. A. Gassman and N. Santoro, "The Influence of Menopausal Hormonal Changes on Sexuality: Current Knowledge and Recommendations for Practice," *Menopause* 1, no. 2 (1994): 91–98.

3. A. Vermuelen and L. Verdonck, "Factors Affecting Sex Hormone Levels in Postmenopausal Women," *Journal of Steroid Biochemistry* 11 (1979): 899–901.

4. R. Azziz and G. Koulianos, "Adrenal Androgens and Reproductive Aging in Females," *Seminar of Reproductive Endocrinology* 9, no. 3 (1991): 249–60.

5. L. Dennerstein, G. Burrows, C. Wood et al., "Hormones and Sexuality: Effect of Estrogen and Progesterone," *Obstetrics and Gynecology* 56, no. 3 (1980): 316–22.

6. Gassman and Santoro, "The Influence of Menopausal Hormonal Changes on Sexuality," 91–97.

7. E. Goldman, "Ginkgo Eases Medication-Induced Sex Dysfunction," *OB.GYN. News* (July 15, 1997): 19.

8. E. S. Johnson et al., "Efficacy of Feverfew as Prophylactic Treatment of Migraine," *British Medical Journal* 291 (1985): 569–73.

CHAPTER 11: *JOINT PAIN AND OSTEOPOROSIS*

1. E. G. Lufkin and M. Zilkoski, "Diagnosis and Management of Osteoporosis," *American Family Physician Monograph.* no. 1 (1996): 3.

2. C. Cooper, G. Campion, and L. J. Melton III, "Hip Fractures in the Elderly: A Worldwide Projection," *Osteoporosis International* 2 (1992): 285–89.

3. L. V. Avioli, *The Osteoporotic Syndrome: Detection, Prevention, and Management,* 3d ed. (New York: Wiley-Liss, 1993), 152.

4. Lufkin and Zilkoski, "Diagnosis and Management of Osteoporosis," 5.

5. C. Kilgore, "Watch Rapid Bone Loss with Glucocorticoid Use," *OB.GYN. News* (August 1, 1997): 8.

6. M. A. Liebert, "Reduced Bone Mass in Women with Premenstrual Syndrome," *Journal of Women's Health* 4, no. 2 (1995): 161–68.

7. S. R. Cummings, D. M. Black, M. C. Nevitt et al., "Bone Density at Various Sites for Prediction of Hip Fractures: The Study of Osteoporotic Fractures Research Group," *Lancet* 34, no. 8837 (1993): 72–75.

8. C. Christiansen, "Does Calcium Supplementation Prevent Postmenopausal Bone Loss? A Double-blind, Controlled Clinical Study," *New England Journal of Medicine* 316 (1987): 173–77.

Greendale et al., "Lifestyle and Bone Density in Women," *Journal of Women's Health* 4, no. 3 (1995): 239.

9. B. Ettinger, *Annals of Internal Medicine* (March 1985).

10. T. J. Garnett, J. W. W. Studd, N. R. Watson, and M. Savvas, "A Cross-sectional Study of the Effects of Long-term Percutaneous Hormone Replacement Therapy on Bone Density," *Obstetrics and Gynecology* 78 (1991): 1002–7.

11. B. Ettinger and D. Grady, "Estrogen Therapy for Osteoporosis," *Menopause* 1, no. 1 (1994): 19–24.

12. H. Daniell, "Menopause and Dental Health," *Menopause Management* 5, no. 1 (1996): 10–11, 24.

13. A. Paganini-Hill, "The Benefits of Estrogen Replacement Therapy on Oral Health," *Archives of Internal Medicine* 155 (1995): 2325.

14. K. Overgaard, R. Lindsay, and C. Christiansen, "Patient Responsiveness to Calcitonin Salmon Nasal Spray: A Subanalysis of a 2-year Study," *Clinical Therapeutics* 17, no. 4, Excerta Medica (1995): 17.

CHAPTER 12: *CARDIOVASCULAR PROBLEMS*

1. K. Newman and J. Sullivan, "Coronary Heart Disease in Women: Epidemiology," *Clinical Syndromes and Management* 3, no. 1 (1996): 51–59.

2. NBC News medical segment, August 19, 1996.

3. B. E. Henderson, A. Paganini-Hill, and R. K. Ross, "Decreased Morbidity in Users of Estrogen Replacement Therapy," *Archives of Internal Medicine* 151 (1991): 75–78.

4. M. J. Stampfer, G. A. Colditz, W. C. Willet et al., "Postmenopausal Estrogen Therapy and Cardiovascular Disease: Ten-year Follow-up from the Nurses' Health Study," *New England Journal of Medicine* 325 (1991): 756–62.

5. Stampfer et al., "Postmenopausal Estrogen Therapy and Cardiovascular Disease," 756–62.

6. *U.S. Mortality Data Tapes, 1968 to 1983* (U.S. Department of Health and Human Services, National Center for Health Statistics, 1984).

7. E. Barrett-Conner and T. L. Bush, "Estrogen and Coronary Heart Disease in Women," *Journal of the American Medical Association* 265 (1991): 1861–67.

Stampfer et al., "Postmenopausal Estrogen Therapy and Cardiovascular Disease," 756–62.

CHAPTER 13: *WELLNESS EATING*

1. B. Sears, *The Zone* (San Francisco: HarperCollins, 1995), 30.

2. J. Haarbo, U. Marslew, A. Gotfredsen et al., "Postmenopausal Hormone Replacement Therapy Prevents Central Distribution of Body Fat after Menopause," *Metabolism* 40 (1991): 1323–26.

J. C. Stevenson, D. Crook, E. F. Godsland et al., "Hormone Replacement Therapy and the Cardiovascular System," *Drugs* 47, suppl. 2 (1994): 23–26.

3. Haarbo et al., "Postmenopausal Hormone Replacement Therapy," 1323–26.

4. Sears, *The Zone*.

A simplified version of "the zone" concept that focuses on the diet rather than the science has been helpful to our patients. It is Joyce and Gene Daoust, *40/30/30 Fat Burning Nutrition: The Dietary, Hormonal Connection to Permanent Weight Loss and Better Health* (Del Mar, Calif.: Wharton, 1996).

5. Snacks that are 30 percent protein, 40 percent carbohydrates, and 30 percent fat are beginning to appear on the market. Please note these are not to be confused with "power bars" that are high in carbohydrates. In our office, because we work with midlife women, we carry a version of bars sold only through physicians because of the addition of GLA, a substance helpful in relieving aches and pains, among other things. Dr. Sears has a line of zone-perfect nutrition bars available. Call 800-233-3426. Anyone who is diabetic or hypoglycemic benefits greatly from having such snacks available. Other brands that we have found adequate if not as tasty or long-lasting are: Biozone Bars (603-598-6289), PR Bar (800-456-1822), EZ 40-30-30 Nutrition (619-439-7552), and Balance Bars (very inexpensive at Trader Joe's stores).

6. Sears, *The Zone*, 11.

7. D. Horrobin et al., "Omega-6 Fatty Acids May Reverse Carcinogenesis by Restoring Natural PGE–1 Metabolism," *Medical Hypothesis* 6 (1980): 469–86.

J. J. Jarkowski and W. T. Cave, "Dietary Fish Oil May Inhibit Development of Breast Cancer," *Journal of the National Cancer Institute* 74 (1985): 1145–50.

8. B. Jancin, "The Skinny on Middle-Age Weight Gain," *OB.GYN. News* (January 1, 1996): 20.

9. A. Brzezinski and J. Wurtman, "Managing Weight through the Transition Years," *Menopause Management* 2, no. 10 (November/December 1993): 18–23.

10. B. Larson, C. Bengtsson, P. Bjorntorp et al., "Is Abdominal Body Fat Distribution a Major Explanation for the Sex Difference in the Incidence of Myocardial Infarction?" *American Journal of Epidemiology* 135 (1992): 266–73.

11. B. Jancin, "High-Soy Diet May Reduce Breast Cancer," *OB.GYN. News* 32, no. 12 (June 15, 1997): 21.

12. A. Brezinski, H. Adlercreutz, R. Shaoul et al., "Short-term Effects of Phytoestrogen-rich Diet on Postmenopausal Women," *Menopause* 4, no. 2 (1997), 88–94.

13. B. L. Smith, "Organic Foods vs. Supermarket Foods: Element Levels," *Journal of Applied Nutrition* 45 (1993): 35–39.

14. "Coverage of Alternative Medicine on the Rise," *OB.GYN. News* (May 15, 1997): 37.

15. J. Charnow, "Selenium Reportedly Lowers Risk of Some Cancers," *Medical Tribune Primary Care* (Feb. 6, 1997): 18; reporting on research findings in the *Journal of the American Medical Association* 276 (1996): 1957–63.

16. S. Boschert, "Increasing Folic Acid Intake Could Benefit Everyone," *OB.GYN. News* (July 15, 1997): 28.

17. M. Percival, "The Importance of Optimal Nutrition," *Clinical Nutrition Insights* 5, no. 3 (1997): 1–6.

18. For those patients who have not been impressed with over-the-counter vitamins, we order multivitamins from Metagenics, a company we have come to trust (800-692-9400). Their commitment is to use natural, high quality ingredients and to rely on sound research.

19. S. N. Meydani, "Vitamin E May Enhance Immune Response in Elderly," *Journal of the American Medical Association* 277 (1997): 1380–86.

20. P. D. Saltman and L. G. Strause, "The Role of Trace Minerals in Osteoporosis," *Journal of the American College of Nutrition* 12, no. 4 (1993): 384–89.

21. J. H. Beattie and H. S. Peace, "The Influence of a Low-boron Diet and Boron Supplementation on Bone, Major Mineral and Sex Steroid Metabolism in Post-menopausal Women," *British Journal of Nutrition* 69 (1993): 871–84.

CHAPTER 14: *WELLNESS MOVING*

1. S. J. Petruzello, D. M. Landers, B. D. Hatfield et al., "A Meta-Analysis on the Anxiety-Reducing Effects of Acute and Chronic Exercise," *Sports Medicine* 11 (1991): 143–82.

2. M. Hammar, J. Brynhildsen et al., "The Effects of Physical Activity on Menopausal Symptoms and Metabolic Changes around Menopause," *Menopause* 2, no. 4 (1995): 201–9.

3. T. L. Schwenk, "Exercise for the Depressed Menopausal Patient," *Menopause Management* (September/October 1995): 14–19.

4. "Exercise Lengthens Life Span for Older Women," *The Female Patient* 22 (July 1997): 76 (from a report in *Journal of the American Medical Association* 277 [1997]: 1287–92).

5. L. Thune, "Regular Exercise May Reduce Risk of Breast Cancer," *New England Journal of Medicine* 336 (1997): 1269–75.

6. Petruzello et al., "A Meta-Analysis on the Anxiety-Reducing Effects of Acute and Chronic Exercise," 143–82.

7. S. L. Wolf, "Tai Chi Helps the Elderly Maintain Their Balance," *Journal of the American Geriatric Society* 44 (1996): 489–97.

CHAPTER 15: *WELLNESS THINKING*

1. D. Mann, "Mental Stress Testing Identifies Those at Risk for Cardiac Events," *Medical Tribune Primary Care* 3, no. 13 (July 18, 1996): 18. Report on the article appeared in the *Journal of the American Medical Association* 275 (1996): 1651–56.

2. D. L. Childre, *Freeze Frame: Fast Action Stress Relief* (Boulder Creek, Calif.: Planetary Publications, 1994), 18.

3. G. Rein, M. Atkinson, and R. McCraty, "The Physiological and Psychological Effects of Compassion and Anger," *Journal of Advancement in Medicine* 8, no. 2 (summer 1995): 87–105.

4. Childre, *Freeze Frame*, 41–42.

5. For information on training programs contact the Institute of HeartMath at 408-338-8700. Their 400–page website is full of science papers, case studies, and descriptions of their programs. You can find them at http//www.webcom.com/hrt math.

6. "Spirituality Is an Often Untapped Resource," *OB.GYN. News* (February 1, 1996): 41.

7. D. B. Larson, *The Faith Factor—Volume Two: An Annotated Bibliography of Systematic Reviews and Clinical Research on Spiritual Subjects* (Rockville, Md.: National Institute for Healthcare Research, 1995).

8. L. Dossey, *Healing Words: The Power of Prayer and the Practice of Medicine* (San Francisco: HarperSanFrancisco, 1993).

9. Thomas Moore, *Care of the Soul* (N.Y.: HarperCollins, 1992).

CHAPTER 16: *THE LESSER-KNOWN OPTIONS*

1. R. S. McCaleb, "Food Ingredients Safety Evaluation," *Food and Drug Law Journal* 4 (1992): 657–65.

2. E. M. Duker et al., "Effects of Extracts from Cimicifuga Racemosa on Gonadotropin Release in Menopausal Women and Ovariectomized Rats," *Planta Medica* 57 (1991): 420–24.

H. Stolze, "An Alternative to Treat Menopause Complaints," *Gynecology* 3 (1982): 14–16.

G. Warnecke, "Influencing Menopausal Symptoms with a Phytotherapeutic Agent," *Med Welt* 36 (1985): 871–74.

Stoll, "Phytopharmacon Influences Atrophic Vaginal Epithelium," 23–33.

3. P. R. Casson and J. Buster, "DHEA Replacement after Menopause: HRT2000 or Nostrum of the '90s?" *Contemporary OB/GYN* 42, no. 4 (April 1997): 119–33.

4. P. Taelman, J. M. Kaufman, X. Janssens, and A. Vereulen, "Persistence of Increased Bone Resorption and Possible Role of Dehydroepiandrosterone as a Non-Metabolism Determinant in Osteoporotic Women in Late Postmenopause," *Maturitas* 11 (1989): 67–73.

E. Barrett-Conner, K-T. Khaw, and S. S. C. Yen, "A Prospective Study of Dehydroepiandrosterone Sulfate, Mortality, and Cardiovascular Disease, *New England Journal of Medicine* 315 (1986): 1519–24.

5. K. J. Helzlsouer et al., "Relationship of Prediagnostic Serum Levels of Dehydroepiandrosterone and Dehydroepiandrosterone Sulfate to the Risk of Developing Premenopausal Breast Cancer," *Cancer Research* 41 (1981): 3360–63.

6. J. F. Mortola and S. S. C. Yen, "The Effects of Oral Dehydroepiandrosterone on Endocrine-Metabolic Parameters in Postmenopausal Women," *Journal of Clinical Endocrinology Metabolism* 71 (1990): 696–704.

7. C. Johannes et al., "The Effect of the Menopausal Transition and Aging on DHEAS Levels in Women," *Menopause* 3, no. 4 (1996): 222.

8. S. E. Monroe and K. M. J. Menon, "Changes in Reproductive Hormone Secretion during the Climacteric and Postmenopausal Periods," *Journal of Clinical Obstetrics and Gynecology* 20 (1977): 113–22. There is a small group of people who have a genetic factor that impairs breakdown of various androgens, and this skews the range somewhat. For women, normal will lie somewhere between 350 and 2,000 micrograms per deciliter, for men, 800 and 3,000 micrograms per deciliter. In one study premenopausal women had an average DHEA level of 542 (ng/100ml), which dropped to 197 for postmenopausal women, and to 126 in women whose ovaries had been surgically removed.

9. B. E. C. Nordin, A. Robertson, R. F. Seamark et al., "The Relationship between Calcium Absorption, Serum Dehydroepiandrosterone, and Vertebral Mineral Density in Postmenopausal Women," *Journal of Clinical Endocrinology Metabolism* 60 (1985): 651–57.

10. Roa-Pena et al., "Immunoreactive Aromatase in Human Bone Cells," *Menopause* 1, no. 2 (1994): 73–77.

11. B. Dobay et al., "Improved Menopausal Symptom Relief with Estrogen-Androgen Therapy," *Menopause* 3, no. 4 (1996), 233.

12. R. Young, "Androgens in Postmenopausal Therapy?" *Menopause Management* (May 1993): 21–24.

13. R. D. Gambrell Jr., "Androgen Therapy," in *Managing the Menopause: An Update*, ed. R. D. Gambrell Jr. (New York: McGraw-Hill, 1989), 11–16.

337

CHAPTER 17: *USE OF NATURAL AND SYNTHETIC ESTROGEN AND PROGESTERONE*

1. P. K. Mansfield and A. M. Voda, "Hormone Use Among Middle-Aged Women," *Menopause* 1, no. 2 (1994): 99–108.

2. B. Baker, "Hormone Therapy Costs Less than Screening," *OB.GYN. News* (December 15, 1995): 9.

3. Personal conversation with Leon Speroff, M.D., August 1996. Dr. Speroff is professor of obstetrics and gynecology, Oregon Health Sciences, University of Portland, and a researcher in women's endocrinology.

4. G. N. Hortobagy, V. Hug, A. U. Buzdar et al., "Sequential Cyclic Combined Hormonal Therapy for Metastatic Breast Cancer," *Cancer* 64 (1989): 1002–6.

5. S. Harlap, "The Benefits and Risks of Hormone Replacement Therapy: An Epidemiologic Overview," *American Journal of Obstetrics and Gynecology* 166 (1992): 1986–92.

6. R. D. Gorsky, J. P. Koplan, H. B. Peterson et al., "Relative Risks and Benefits of Long-Term Estrogen Replacement Therapy: A Decision Analysis," *Obstetrics and Gynecology* 83 (1994): 161–66.

7. R. Wild, "Estrogen: Effects on the Cardiovascular Tree," *Obstetrics and Gynecology* 87 (1996): 27s–35s.

8. Writing Group for the PEPI Trial, "Effects of Estrogen or Estrogen/Progestin Regimens on Heart Disease Factors in Postmenopausal Women: The Postmenopausal Estrogen/Progestin Interventions (PEPI) Trial," *Journal of the American Medical Association* 273 (1990): 287–98.

9. K. Thornton, "Glucose Metabolism: Effects of HRT," *Menopause Management* 15, no. 2 (May/June 1996): 21–26.

10. B. McEwen, "Estrogens and Neuronal Connectivity and Viability" (paper presented at North American Menopause Society annual meeting, San Diego, Calif., September 4, 1993).

11. P. M. Sarrel, "Ovarian Hormones and the Circulation," *Maturitas* 12 (1990): 287–98.

12. J. M. Sullivan, A. Bashar et al., "Progestin Enhances Vasoconstrictor Responses in Postmenopausal Women Receiving Estrogen Replacement Therapy," *Menopause* 2, no. 4 (1995): 193–99.

13. M. Penotti et al., "Long-term Effects of Postmenopausal Hormone Replacement Therapy on Pulsatility Index of Internal Carotid and Middle Cerebral Arteries," *Menopause* 4, no. 2 (1997), 101–4.

14. J. K. Keaney, G. T. Scwairy, A. Xu et al., "17B-Estradiol Preserves Endothelial Vasodilator Function and Limits Low-density Lipoprotein Oxidation in Hypercholesterolemic Swine," *Circulation* 89 (1994): 2251–59.

15. G. Grodstein et al., "Postmenopausal Hormone Therapy and Mortality," *New England Journal of Medicine* 336 (1997): 1769–75.

16. N. Panay and J. Studd, "Progestogen/Progesterone and Bone Loss," *Menopause* 3, no. 1 (1996): 13–19.

17. M. Gelfand, P. Fugere, F. Wiita et al., "Conjugated Estrogens Combined with Sequential Dydrogesterone or Medroxyprogesterone Acetate in Postmenopausal Women," *Menopause* 4, no. 1 (1997): 10–18.

18. R. D. Gambrell Jr., "Estrogen Replacement Therapy and Breast Cancer Risk: A New Look at the Data," *Female Patient* 18 (1993): 50–62.

I. Persson, J. Yuen, L. Bergkvist et al., "Combined Oestrogen-Progestogen Replacement and Breast Cancer Risk" (letter), *Lancet* 340 (1992): 1044.

19. J. L. Bullock, F. M. Massey, and R. D. Gambrell, "Use of Medroxyprogesterone Acetate to Prevent Menopausal Symptoms," *Obstetrics and Gynecology* 46 (1975): 165–68.

20. J. C. Prior, "Progesterone as a Bone-Tropic Hormone," *Endocrinology Review* 11 (1990): 386–98.

21. K. Dalton and M. J. T. Dalton, "DPMA and Bone Density," *British Medical Journal* 303 (1991): 855.

22. Panay and Studd, "Progestogen/Progesterone and Bone Loss," 13–19.

23. Prior, "Progesterone as a Bone-Tropic Hormone," 386–98.

R. A. Lobo, "The Role of Progestins in Hormone Replacement Therapy," *American Journal of Obstetrics and Gynecology* 166 (1990): 1997–2004.

24. N. Panay and J. Studd, "Do Progestogens and Progesterone Reduce Bone Loss?" *Journal of the North American Menopause Society* 3, no. 1 (1996): 13–19.

25. S. Dentali, "The American Herb Association," 10, no. 1 (1995): 4.

The wild yam contains the phytosteroid diosgenin, which is the starting point in the chemical manufacturing process of progesterone. In soybeans the process begins with stigmasterol from which genistein is derived.

CHAPTER 18: *LOOKING AT THE BONUSES*

1. P. A. Newcomb, "Menopausal Hormone Use and Risk of Large-Bowel Cancer," *Journal of the National Cancer Institute* 87 (July 1995): 1067–95.

2. D. Alberts, "Randomized, Double-Blinded, Placebo-Controlled Study of Effect of Wheat Bran Fiber and Calcium on Fecal Bile Acids in Patients with Resected Adenomatous Colon Polyps," *Journal of the National Cancer Institute* 88 (1996): 81–92.

3. V. W. Henderson, A. Paganini-Hill, C. K. Emanuel et al., "Estrogen Replacement Therapy in Older Women: Comparisons between Alzheimer's Disease Cases and Non-demented Controls," *Archives of Neurology* 51 (1994): 896–901.

T. Ohkura et al., "Low-Dose ERT for Alzheimer's Disease," *Menopause* 1, no. 3 (1994): 125–30.

4. M. Johnson, "Estrogen May Cut Risk of Alzheimer's, Study Finds," *The Press Democrat* (Santa Rosa, Calif.), 16 August 1996, A6.

5. A. Paganini-Hill and V. W. Henderson, "Estrogen Deficiency and Risk of Alzheimer's Disease in Women," *American Journal of Epidemiology* 140 (1994): 256.

6. S. M. Phillips and B. B. Sherwin, "Effects of Estrogen on Memory Function in Surgically Menopausal Women," *Psychoneuroendocrinology* 17 (1992): 485.

D. L. Kampen and B. B. Sherwin, "Estrogen Use and Verbal Memory in Healthy Postmenopausal Women," *Obstetrics and Gynecology* 83 (1994): 979.

7. L. Speroff and V. W. Henderson, "Estrogen: Does It Lower the Risk for Alzheimer's?" *Contemporary OB/GYN* 41, no. 5 (1996): 133–42.

8. R. D. Brinton, "Estrogen Replacement Therapy and Alzheimer's Disease," *Menopausal Medicine* 5, no. 1 (spring 1997): 5–8.

9. J. Kahn, "Type I Diabetes Linked with Early Menopause," *Medical Tribune* (July 17, 1997): 16.

CHAPTER 19: *CHECKING OUT THE FINE PRINT*

1. M. Coyle and B. Panchmatia, "Women's Reasons for and Barriers to Seeking Care for Breast Cancer Symptoms," *Women's Health Issues* 5, no. 1 (spring 1995): 27–35.

2. R. Sands et al., "HRT and Breast Cancer Symptoms," *Women's Health Issues* 5, no. 2 (1995): 73–80.

3. J. Stenson, "High-Fat Diet May Not Increase Breast-Cancer Link," *Medical Tribune Oncology* 13, no. 11 (1996): 4.

4. J. Cuzick, D. K. Wong, and R. D. Bulbrook, "The Prevention of Breast Cancer," *Lancet* i (1986): 83–86.

5. J. A. Horton, ed., *The Women's Health Data Book*, 2d ed. (Washington, D.C.: The Jacobs Institute of Women's Health, 1995): 64.

6. B. A. Miller, L. A. G. Ries, B. F. Hankey, et al., *Seer Cancer Statistics Review: 1973–1990* (Bethesda, Md.: National Cancer Institute, 1993, NIH publication no. 93-2789).

7. "Exploring the Link between Birth Weight and Later Breast Cancer," *OBGYN Management* (July 1997), 35.

8. N. Childs, "Regular Exercise May Reduce Risk of Breast Cancer," *OB.GYN. News* 32, no. 12 (June 15, 1997): 4.

9. Seminar materials, University of San Francisco Continuing Medical Education, Palm Drive Hospital, Sebastopol, Calif., July 1996.

10. J. Kluger, "Cancer Genes Revisited," *Time* (May 26, 1997): 70.

11. B. Jancin, "Prophylactic Mastectomy Cuts Risk by 91 Percent," *OB.GYN. News* 32, no. 12 (June 15, 1997): 17.

12. J. S. O'Neill, W. R. Miller, et al., "Breast Cyst Fluid Concentrations of Beta Endorphin, Steroids, and Gonadotrophins in Premenopausal Women with Gross Cystic Disease," *Maturitas* 13 (1991): 123–28.

13. J. C. Arpels and R. D. Nachtigall, "Gonadal Hormones and Breast Cancer Risk," *Menopause* 1, no. 1 (1994): 49–55.

14. A. Spira, "The Decline of Fecundity with Age," *Maturitas*, suppl. 1 (1988): 15–22.

15. C. Malet, A. Gompel, A. Vaneva et al., "Estradiol and Progesterone Receptors in Cultured Normal Human Breast Epithelial Cells and Fibroblasts: Immunocytochemical Studies," *Clinical Endocrinology Metabolism* 73 (1991): 8–17.

16. W. D. Dupont and D. L. Page, "Menopausal Estrogen Replacement Therapy and Breast Cancer," *Archives of Internal Medicine* 151 (1991): 57–72.

K. K. Steinberg, S. B. Thacker, S. J. Smith et al., "A Meta-Analysis of the Effect of Estrogen Replacement Therapy on the Risk of Breast Cancer," *Journal of the American Medical Association* 265 (1991): 1985–90.

17. D. Mann, "HRT Prolongs Most Women's Lives Study Concludes," *Medical Tribune* 4, no. 5 (May 1, 1997): 1. Summary of HRT report in the *Journal of the American Medical Association* 277 (1997): 1140–47.

18. I. Bergkvist, H. Adami, I. Persson et al., "The Risk of Breast Cancer after Estrogen and Estrogen-Progestin Replacement," *New England Journal of Medicine* 321 (1989): 293–97.

19. L. Speroff, "Postmenopausal Hormone Therapy and Breast Cancer," *Obstetrics and Gynecology* 87, no. 2, suppl. (February 1996): 44s–54s.

20. G. A. Colditz, S. E. Hankinson, D. J. Hunter et al., "The Use of Estrogens and Progestins and the Risk of Breast Cancer in Postmenopausal Women," *New England Journal of Medicine* 332, no. 24 (June 15, 1995): 1589–93.

21. I. Bergkvist, H. O. Adami, I. Persson et al., "Prognosis after Breast Cancer Diagnosis in Women Exposed to Estrogen and Estrogen-Progestogen Replacement Therapy," *American Journal of Epidemiology* 130 (1992): 221–28.

22. S. Boschert, "Survey Shows ERT Protects against Breast Cancer Death," *OB.GYN. News* 31, no. 11 (1996): 1–2.

23. W. D. Dupont, D. L. Page, L. W. Rogers et al., "Influence of Exogenous Estrogens on Proliferative Breast Disease," *New England Journal of Medicine* 63 (1989): 948.

24. W. H. Hindle, "The Continuing Controversy about Breast Cancer Risk and Estrogen Replacement Therapy," *Menopause Management* (September/October 1995): 12–13.

25. Colditz et al., "The Use of Estrogens and Progestins and the Risk of Breast Cancer in Postmenopausal Women," 1589–93.

26. P. N. Matthews, R. R. Millis, and J. L. Haywood, "Breast Cancer in Women Who Have Taken Contraceptive Steroids," *British Medical Journal* 282 (1981): 774–76.

27. J. L. Stanford, "Combined Estrogen and Progestin Hormone Replacement Therapy in Relation to Risk of Breast Cancer in Middle-aged Women," *Journal of the American Medical Association* 274 (July 12, 1995): 137–42.

28. Bergkvist et al., "Prognosis after Breast Cancer Diagnosis in Women Exposed to Estrogen and Estrogen-Progestogen Replacement Therapy," 221–28.

29. B. K. Armstrong, "Oestrogen Therapy after the Menopause—Boon or Ban?" *Medical Journal of Australia* 148 (1988): 213–14.

Dupont and Page, "Menopausal Estrogen Replacement Therapy and Breast Cancer," 67–72.

Steinberg et al., "A Meta-Analysis of the Effect of Estrogen Replacement Therapy on the Risk of Breast Cancer," 1985–90.

M. Sillero-Arenas, M. Delgado-Rodriquez, R. Rodriquez-Canteras et al., "Menopausal Hormone Replacement Therapy and Breast Cancer: A Meta-Analysis," *Obstetrics and Gynecology* 79 (1992): 286–94.

G. A. Colditz, K. M. Egan, and M. J. Stamfer, "Hormone Replacement Therapy and Risk of Breast Cancer: Results from Epidemiologic Studies," *American Journal of Obstetrics and Gynecology* 168 (1993): 1473–80.

K. K. Steinberg, S. J. Smith, S. B. Thacker et al., "Breast Cancer Risk and Duration of Estrogen Use: The Role of Study Design in Meta-Analysis," *Epidemiology* 5 (1994): 415–21.

J. A. Roy, C. A. Sawka, and K. I. Pritchard, "Hormone Replacement Therapy in Women with Breast Cancer: Do the Risks Outweigh the Benefits?" *Journal of Clinical Oncology* 14, no. 3 (1996): 997–1006.

30. D. M. Strickland, R. D. Gambrell Jr., C. A. Butzin et al., "The Relationship between Breast Cancer Survival and Prior Postmenopausal Estrogen Use," *Obstetrics and Gynecology* 80 (1992): 400–404.

31. P. J. DiSaia, F. Odicino, E. A. Grosen et al., "Hormone Replacement Therapy in Breast Cancer," *Lancet* 342 (1993): 1232.

A. Eden, T. Bush, S. Nand, and B. G. Wren, "The Royal Hospital for Women's Breast Cancer Study—A Case-controlled Study of Combined, Continuous Oestrogen-Progestogen Replacement Therapy amongst Women with a Personal History of Breast Cancer," submitted to *Obstetrics and Gynecology,* 1995.

32. J. A. Eden, T. Bush, S. Nand, and B. Wren, "A Case-control Study of Combined, Continuous Estrogen Progestin Replacement Therapy among Women with a Personal History of Breast Cancer," *Menopause* 2, no. 2 (1995): 67.

P. DiSaia, "Hormone Replacement Therapy in Breast Cancer Patients," *Contemporary OB/GYN* 41, no. 4 (1996): 67-72, 82-84.

33. M. Jager, S. Kramer, and M. Lang, "Disseminated Breast Cancer: Does Early Treatment Prolong Survival without Symptoms?" *(Lancet* Conference, Bruges, Belgium, April 21-22, 1994), 54.

34. B. G. Wren and J. A Eden, "Progestogens and Breast Cancer," *Menopause* 3, no. 1 (1996): 7.

35. R. A. Badwe, W. M. Gregory, M. A. Chaundary et al., "Timing of Surgery during Menstrual Cycle and Survival of Premenopausal Women with Operable Breast Cancer," *Lancet* 337 (1991): 1261-64.

36. H. Voherr, "Oral Contraceptives and Hormone Replacement Therapy: Are Progestogens and Progestins Breast Mitogens?" *American Journal of Obstetrics and Gynecology* 155 (1986): 1140-42.

CHAPTER 20: MENOPAUSE IMPOSTORS

1. J. Stenson, "Unrecognized Thyroid Disorders on the Rise," *Medical Tribune Primary Care* (February 8, 1996): 9.

2. Symptoms of hypothyroidism were adapted from "Unmasking the *Hidden* Health Problem," from Knoll Pharmaceutical Company, 3000 Continental Drive North, Mount Olive, NJ 07828-1234.

3. Adapted from *Role of Androgens in Menopause,* Georgetown University School of Medicine Continuing Medical Education Program booklet, sponsored by Solvay Pharmaceuticals, January 15, 1996, 8.

4. The Adrenal Stress Index is a product of Diagnos-techs, Inc., a federally regulated and licensed laboratory (CLIA license 50DO630141) 6620 S. 192nd Pl., #J-104, Kent, WA 98032, 206-251-0596 or 1-800-87-TESTS.

5. R. Inman, "Rheumatic Disease," *Clinicians of North America* 17, no. 2 (1991): 309-21.

6. Metagenics Headquarters, 971 Calle Negocio, San Clemente, CA 92673, 800-692-9400. Metagenics Northern California, 130 Ryan Court, #200, San Ramon, CA 94583, 510-838-7858 or 800-334-1700. Patients sensitive to the FOS in Ultra Flora should substitute Ultra Dophilus and Ultra Bifidus separately.

7. InterPlexus, Inc., P.O. Box 58948, Seattle, WA 98138-1948, 800-875-0511.

8. J. S. Bland, *The 20-Day Rejuvenation Diet Program* (New Canaan, Conn.: Keats Publishing, 1977). Dr. Bland has been actively involved in nutrition-related research for twenty years and has served as director of the Bellevue-Redmond Medical Laboratory. He is founder of HealthComm, Inc., a leading research and development company in the field of functional medicine.

9. The products we use that were developed by Dr. Bland are from Metagenics: UltraClear Plus, UltraClear, and UltraSustain. Dr. Bland's book tells how to use diet alone to improve liver and gut health.

10. J. Bland, May 13, 1997, Gig Harbor, Washington, press release. "Health-Comm International, Inc., announces patent issue for premier metabolic detoxifi-

cation product, UltraClear." HealthComm International, Inc., P.O. Box 1729, Gig Harbor, WA 98335, 206-851-3943.

11. The 4-R Gastrointestinal Support Plan was developed by scientists at Health-Comm International, Inc., U.S. patent #5, 629, 023, under the direction of Dr. Jeffrey Bland. It is available exclusively from Metagenics, 800-692-9400.

APPENDIX A: QUESTIONS AND ANSWERS

1. C. B. Coulam et al., "Incidence of Premature Ovarian Failure," *American Journal of Obstetrics and Gynecology* 67, no. 4 (1986): 27.

2. J. E. Hade and H. Spiro, "Calcium and Acid Rebound: A Reappraisal," *Journal of Clinical Gastroenterology* 15, no. 1 (1992): 37–44.

3. Whitlock et al., "Prevalence of HRT Contraindications," *Journal of Women's Health* 4, no. 3 (June 1995): 279.

Index

A Woman's Place, located in Northern California's tranquil Sonoma County, provides medically sound, balanced evaluations of each woman's unique response to midlife and the menopausal passage. Should you wish to contact the Mayos, please use the following information:

Joseph L. Mayo, M.D., FACOG
Mary Ann Mayo, M.A., MFT
P.O. Box 1039
Geyserville, CA 95441
Ph. 800-750-2568; 707-431-0117
Fax: 707-431-8126
http://www.menopausemanager.com

Mary Ann Mayo, M.A., MFT, and Joseph L. Mayo, M.D., FACOG, Stanford-trained OB/GYN, are partners in the goal of promoting the wellness of women in midlife. Cofounders of A Woman's Place Medical Center in Healdsburg, California, they have employed an integrative approach to their patients' problems, combining alternative and conventional therapies as appropriate. Currently they are speaking nationally on women's health.

Mary Ann Mayo is the author of eight books that address women's mental and physical health. She has appeared on *The Oprah Winfrey Show* and has written about health for a number of national magazines and a newletter. She is a charter member of the Educational Affiliates of the American College of Obstetrics and Gynecology.

Dr. Joseph Mayo has been a dedicated practitioner of women's health for more than twenty-five years. He is a fellow of the American College of Obstetrics and Gynecology.

The Mayos are both members of the North American Menopause Society. They have been married for thirty-seven years.